Private Health Sector Growth in Asia

DEDICATION

This book is dedicated to the memory of James R. Jeffers, 1938 to 1996, one of the contributors to this book. Jim was an important member of the ten-member team assembled by Management Sciences for Health to work on the Asian Development Bank's Second Regional Conference on Health Sector Reform in March 1996, which was the basis for this book. He died of a heart attack in Cairo on 15 June 1996 and is survived by his wife Somkit, who resides in Chiang Mai, Thailand.

Jim was a superb technician as a health economist, and a kind and generous human being. He grew up on a farm in Iowa, graduated from the University of Iowa, and received a PhD in economics from Tulane University. Professionally, Jim started as a health economist working in the USA at the University of Iowa, where he served as a professor for over 20 years. He was a pioneer in the development of the discipline of the economics of health care and founded the Health Economics Research Center in the College of Business Administration at the University. In the 1980s he began working internationally. He worked as a health economist in over 20 countries, including Malaysia, Indonesia, Korea, Thailand, the Philippines, Kenya and Egypt.

Until last year, he served as Health Economist on the Philippines Health Finance Development Project managed by Management Sciences for Health, which worked with the Government of the Philippines to improve the financing of health services. One of Jim's enduring legacies is his instrumental advisory role in developing the concept, drafting the legislation, and seeing the passage of the National Health Insurance Law in the Philippines in 1995.

In preparing this book, Jim was of great help to the editor and the other contributors. He assisted by traveling to the various study countries with the editor to provide technical support to the research process. His insights, intensity, advice and humor were valued by all. His friends and colleagues alike around the world will miss him sorely.

Private Health Sector Growth in Asia

Issues and Implications

Edited by

WILLIAM NEWBRANDER

Management Sciences for Health, Boston, USA

JOHN WILEY & SONS

Chichester · New York · Weinheim · Brisbane · Singapore · Toronto

Chapters 2, 3, 5, 8 and 11 reprinted with corrections from *The International Journal of Health Planning and Management*, **11**(3):203–296 (1996). Copyright © 1996 John Wiley & Sons Ltd

Other Wiley Editorial Offices

John Wiley & Sons, Inc., 605 Third Avenue, New York, NY 10158-0012, USA

VCH Verlagsgesellschaft, Pappelallee 3, D-69469 Weinheim, Germany

Jacaranda Wiley Ltd, 33 Park Road, Milton, Queensland 4064, Australia

John Wiley & Sons (Asia) Pte Ltd, Clementi Loop #02-01, Jin Xing Distripark, Singapore 129809

John Wiley & Sons (Canada) Ltd, 22 Worcester Road, Rexdale, Ontario M9W 1L1, Canada

Library of Congress Cataloging-in-Publication Data

Private health sector growth in Asia / edited by William Newbrander.
     p. cm.
    "Asian Development Bank's (ADB) Second Regional Conference on
Health Sector Reform: issues related to private sector growth, RETA
5614 held at the Bank in Manila, 5 to 7 March 1996"–
–Acknowledgements.
    Contains five chapters previously published as an issue of
the International journal of health planning and management, July
–Sept., 1996, v. 11, no. 3.
    Includes bibliographical references and index.
    ISBN 0-471-97236-3 (cased : alk. paper)
    1. Medical care — Asia — Finance — Congresses.   2. Medical care–
–Finance — Government policy — Asia — Congresses. 3. Privatization–
–Congresses.   I. Newbrander, William C.   II. Asian Development
Bank.   III. Asian Development Bank's Regional Conference on Health
Sector Reform (2nd : 1996 : Manila, Philippines)   IV. International
journal of health planning and management.
    [DNLM: 1. Delivery of Health Care — organization & administration–
–Asia — congresses.   2. Privatization — trends — Asia — congresses.
3. Insurance, Health — economics — Asia — congresses.   4. Quality
Assurance, Health Care — Asia — congresses.   W 84 JA1 P9 1997]
RA410.55.A78P75   1997
338.4′33621′095 — DC21
DNLM/DLC
for Library of Congress   96-47180
                                                    CIP

British Library Cataloguing in Publication Data

A catalogue record for this book is available from the British Library

ISBN 0-471-97236-3

Typeset in 10/12pt Times by Dobbie Typesetting, Tavistock, Devon
Printed and bound in Great Britain by Bookcraft (Bath) Ltd.
This book is printed on acid-free paper responsibly manufactured from sustainable forestation, for which at least two trees are planted for each one used for paper production

Contents

PART I   OVERVIEW

Figures

Chapter 9

Tables

Chapter 11

Chapter 12

Contributors

Professor P. Berman *Department of Population and International Health, Harvard School of Public Health, Building 1, Room 1210, 665 Huntingdon Avenue, Boston, Massachusetts 02115, USA.*

Peter Berman has been an Associate Professor at the Harvard School of Public Health since 1991, where he currently works on the Data for Decision Making Project. He also provides consulting on health financing. Former positions include Program Officer at the Ford Foundation and Assistant Professor at Johns Hopkins University. He received his PhD in Economics and Nutrition from Cornell University, New York, USA.

Professor R. Bhat *Associate Professor, Indian Institute of Management, Vestrapur, Ahmedabad, 380 015 Gujarat, India.*

Ramesh Bhat is Professor at the Indian Institute of Management, Ahmedabad. He is coordinator of the Health Policy Development Network (HELPONET) in India, supported by the International Health Policy Program, Washington, DC. He is also Adjunct Professor in the Department of Health Policy and Administration at the University of North Carolina at Chapel Hill and has taught the Health Care Financial Management course in their EPDC Programs. He was a Takemi Fellow at Harvard University. He holds a PhD from the Delhi School of Economics, University of Delhi, India.

Professor P. H. Dung *Center for Social Sciences for Health, 138 Giang VO, Hanoi, Vietnam.*

Pham Huy Dung is a Professor of Public Health with the Hanoi Medical Faculty. He is also Vice Director of the Center for Support of Social Development Programs (Union of Scientific and Technological Societies), a nongovernmental organization, and founder and Vice Director of the Center for Social Sciences for Health. He has studied health sector reform, including the role played by teaching hospitals, and health system research. He received his MD and PhD from Hanoi University.

Professor A. Gani *Dean, School of Public Health, University of Indonesia, Kampus Ui-Depok, Indonesia.*

Ascobat Gani is the Dean of the School of Public Health, University of Indonesia, a position he has held since 1994. He provided consulting services in health economics and health policy before joining the University. He was awarded his MD degree from the University of Indonesia, and went on to obtain an MPH from the University of Hawaii and a DrPH from Johns Hopkins University, Maryland, USA.

Professor A. Herrin *School of Economics, University of the Philippines, Diliman, Quezon City, Manila, Philippines.*

Alejandro Herrin is a Professor in the School of Economics, University of the Philippines. He has worked on the development of national health accounts and researched the private health sector in the Philippines. He received his PhD in Economics from the University of South Carolina, USA.

Dr J. Jeffers *Management Sciences for Health, 165 Allandale Road, Boston, Massachusetts 02130, USA.*

James Jeffers was a consultant with Management Sciences for Health's (MSH) Health Financing Program. He previously worked with MSH in the Philippines, serving as Health Policy Adviser to the Health Finance Development Project; prior to that, he worked in Asia, Africa and Latin America for organizations such as ISTI, Birch & Davis, and Westinghouse Health Systems. He held a PhD in Economics from Tulane University, Louisiana, USA.

Professor D. Mongkolsmai *Assistant Professor, Faculty of Economics, Thammasat University, Bangkok, Thailand.*

Dow Mongkolsmai is an Associate Professor with the Faculty of Economics at Thammasat University in Thailand, where she has been for over 10 years; in addition, she is Director of the Economic Research and Training Center of the University. She has also served as a consultant on the Thai health care industry for private firms and international agencies. She was awarded a PhD in Economics from Cornell University, New York, USA.

Ms P. Moser *Project Economist, Asian Development Bank, Manila, Philippines.*

Patricia Moser has been a Health Economist with the Asian Development Bank since 1995. In addition to managing regional activities in health sector reform, she is working on social sector reform in Mongolia and the Central Asian Republics. She has worked in bilateral and multilateral health finance development initiatives in Latin America and Asia for the past 10 years. She received her Master's degree in Economics from the University of North Carolina, USA.

Dr W. Newbrander *Health Economist, Management Sciences for Health, 165 Allandale Road, Boston, Massachusetts 02130, USA.*

William Newbrander is a Health Economist and Principal Program Associate with MSH Health Financing Program in Boston. Prior to joining MSH, he worked with WHO for 8 years, both as Health Economist at their Geneva headquarters and as Program Management Officer for the WHO offices in Thailand and Papua New Guinea. He has served as a hospital administrator in the United States and other countries. He has authored journal articles and is co-author of the book *Decentralization in a Developing Country: The Experience of Papua New Guinea and its Health Service* and the WHO document *Hospital Economics and Financing in*

Developing Countries. He received his PhD in Health Economics and also earned a Masters of Hospital Administration and Masters of Applied Economics from the University of Michigan, USA.

Dr G. Rosenthal   *Health Economist, Management Sciences for Health, 165 Allandale Road, Boston, Massachusetts 02130, USA.*

Gerald Rosenthal is a Health Economist and Senior Program Associate with the MSH Health Financing Program. He worked at Pathfinder International prior to joining MSH. Internationally, he has served as an adviser to the Mexican Secretariat of Health and as Director of REACH, a global health financing project. He holds a PhD in Economics from Harvard University, Massachusetts, USA.

Professor B.-M. Yang   *School of Public Health, Seoul National University Yunkin-Dong, Chongro-ku, Seoul 118-099, Korea.*

Bong-min Yang has been a Professor at Seoul National University since 1994. He was also a Takemi Fellow at Harvard University. He serves as adviser on health and environmental policy matters to the Government of the Republic of Korea. Professor Yang has been a consultant in health financing for the Asian Development Bank and the World Bank. He was awarded a PhD in Economics from Pennsylvania State University, USA.

Acknowledgements

This collection of papers was prepared for the Asian Development Bank (ADB)'s Second Regional Conference on Health Sector Reform: Issues Related to Private Sector Growth, RETA 5614 held at the Bank in Manila, 5 to 7 March 1996. Management Sciences for Health (MSH) of Boston organized the conference and commissioned these papers under contract COCS no. 95-187 with the ADB.

Both the ADB Regional Conference and publication of this book are a culmination of the efforts of many people. The editor would like to acknowledge the contribution of Dr Jane Thomason, formerly of ADB and now District Manager of Royal Childrens Hospital and District Health Service in Queensland and Associate Professor in the Faculty of Medicine of the University of Queensland, Australia. She identified the need for this conference, formulated the conceptual framework, and provided the initial technical direction. Ms Patricia Moser, ADB Project Economist, was responsible for working with the editor and Management Sciences for Health to organize and manage the Regional Conference. Special thanks are also due Mr William Fraser, Manager of Education, Health and Population Division (East) of the Bank's Agriculture and Social Sectors Department (East) for his unwavering support of the Regional Conference and this publication.

The papers of this book were the result of a year-long effort by the authors, who are thanked for their diligent and dedicated work. They worked as a team to provide their individual and corporate contributions and to lead discussions at the conference. Without their tireless endeavors, the efforts of the others would have been for naught. Dr James Jeffers assisted the editor in reviewing the initial outlines and drafts of these papers. He and the editor traveled to the study countries twice, with the resources provided by the ADB, to support the authors in their gathering of data. A selection of the papers was published as an issue of *The International Journal of Health Planning and Management*, July–September, 1996; Volume 11, No. 3. Many thanks to Kenneth Lee, Editor-in-Chief of the journal, and John Wiley & Sons for allowing the reprint of these papers.

I would also thank Dr Ronald O'Connor, founder and President of MSH, for his support to the editor which ensured the success of the ADB Regional Conference and publication of this book. Sybilla Dorros skilfully revised, refined and edited the papers for the conference and for this publication under extremely tight deadlines. Barbara Timmons of MSH provided the professional support to prepare the papers for final publication. Chris Welch capably handled the creation of the tables and figures for each chapter, made the numerous changes required for the book, and provided the overall logistical coordination of this effort.

Over the past year, the MSH Health Financing Program support staff, Donna Shopel, Liz Lewis and Chris Welch, managed the logistics of this project and the conference, from collecting the drafts from the authors to coordinating conference travel arrangements with participants and the ADB. Kathleen Ella of ADB was instrumental in the successful administrative organization of the conference.

Finally, the views expressed in this collection of papers are those of the authors and do not necessarily represent those of the Asian Development Bank or Management Sciences for Health.

WILLIAM NEWBRANDER
Management Sciences for Health

Part I
Overview

1

Private Health Sector Growth in Asia: An Introduction

WILLIAM NEWBRANDER

Health Economist, Management Sciences for Health

and

PATRICIA MOSER

Project Economist, Asian Development Bank

1.1 BACKGROUND

Asia at the end of the twentieth century is in the midst of an economic, political and social transformation. At midcentury, much of the region was marked by widespread subsistence poverty and low social indicators. Now many of the countries are poised to enter the next century on a rising curve of rapid economic growth and human resource development. Incomes are rising, literacy and education levels are increasing, productive life spans are becoming longer, and mortality and morbidity are decreasing. Access to modern health services and technologies has played an important role in this transformation.

Every country in the region developed, in an earlier period, a publicly-financed delivery system for health services. Recently, however, traditional attitudes about the role of government in financing resources for health have changed. The changing attitudes of policy- and decision-makers, planners and managers have affected long-standing ideological beliefs, political systems, and public institutions. In many countries, government is no longer viewed as the necessary "engine of development" and main provider and financier of health services.

As the economies of Asian countries have matured and an increasing proportion of their gross domestic product is used for health, additional resources have become available. However, government resources have not been sufficient to maintain the existing health systems, to meet increased demand due to population growth and rising public expectations, to increase access to services for those not covered by the current systems, and to improve the quality and level of care provided. Concerns about the ability of governments to finance health services adequately, the poor performance of public health service delivery systems, and the desire to expand the choices available to patients have led a number of countries in Asia to adopt a strategy of encouraging the expansion of the private sector.

Private Health Sector Growth in Asia: Issues and Implications. Edited by W. Newbrander.
© 1997 John Wiley & Sons, Ltd.

Many of these countries have looked to the private sector to fill the resource gap by taking on greater responsibilities. Other countries have sought to privatize the public health system as a way of disengaging the government from the health sector, with its rising costs, public dissatisfaction, and a myriad of other problems. As a result, where allowed by government policy (or lack of policy), the private sector has become a major actor in the health sector. In many countries in Asia, government is no longer the main provider and financier of health services. Thus a role for the private sector in health has begun to evolve, either by design or default.

The countries in Asia have experienced this evolution differently due to their unique historical, cultural, economic and political circumstances. Newbrander and Parker (1992) observed that the roles of the public and private sectors in the financing of health services are related to differences in access to care, the range of health services available, and other political and economic factors. They noted that in 13 Asian countries private sector activity is strong: the private, public and insurance components as a percentage of total health expenditure were 48, 42 and 10 per cent, respectively. In these same countries, private expenditures on health, as a proportion of total health expenditure, ranged from 8 to 71 per cent, with a median of 58 per cent (Griffin, 1992).[1]

Indeed, the strength of private sector activity is evidenced in many developing countries in Asia. For instance, in India, 57 per cent of hospitals and 32 per cent of the beds are private; in the Republic of Korea, the proportion of private hospitals has increased from 35 to 95 per cent in the last 10 years; and in the Philippines, 67 per cent of hospitals are private and account for half of all hospital beds, while in Thailand, only 30 per cent of hospitals are private. In India and Thailand, the share of health expenditures from private sources is around 88 per cent; in Indonesia, 65 per cent; in Korea 60 per cent; in the Philippines, approximately 50 per cent.

As the private sector has grown, government concerns have also evolved to cover more than the adequacy of available resources. The issues countries now seek to include in the debate on the roles of government and the private sector encompass quality, equity, differences in access to care, the scope of health services available, emphasis on personal and hospital care rather than primary and preventive care, and resource allocation. These questions have generated discussion on the role of the public sector in private health care markets.

The primary economic rationale for expanding the role of the private sector in the health system is to promote allocative and productive efficiency. The public sector can finance and provide purely public goods, while the private sector should be encouraged to participate more fully in providing private goods. Where a mix of public and private goods exists, there can be some public/private sector mix. In addition to creating incentives for productive efficiency, it is argued that there will be better allocative efficiency if the private sector provides care for certain groups

---

[1]For 21 African countries, private expenditures on health ranged from 14 to 81 per cent of total health expenditure, with a median of 51 per cent (Akin *et al.*, 1987). By contrast, public spending accounts for more than three-quarters of health spending, on average, in OECD countries and accounts for more than 60 per cent of spending in all countries except the USA and Turkey, where it is above 40 per cent (OECD, 1990).

because doing so will free up resources for the public sector to provide services to the underserved.

While increased private sector provision of health services has the potential to provide high-quality curative services and permits governments to divert their limited resources to improve access and extend coverage of health services to the poor and high-risk groups, there are problems in treating the private sector as just another market. Consumers have insufficient information about quality and about appropriate treatments. They must often rely on providers to act as their agents in making decisions about health care once treatment is initiated. Providers may have incentives to act in ways that may conflict with the best interests of patients.

Private sector growth in health has potential problems as well as possible benefits: the public sector may have to compete with the private sector for scarce resources such as personnel, which may increase costs. The public sector may lose important advocates for maintaining the system as higher- and middle-income groups increasingly use the private sector for their care. The development of a private sector catering to higher-income and urban populations may create two different standards of care. Scarce resources needed for other aspects of national development may be allocated to personal health services.

Private sector growth may also result in changes in the demand side of the health system, that is, the financing of health services. Health insurance schemes may proliferate. Various forms of social, private and employer-based health insurance have become common throughout Asia. Thailand passed a social security act in 1990 that included health insurance. The Philippines passed a national health insurance act in 1995, while Korea has had insurance since 1977. Such legislation may result in increased utilization of the private sector, because it reduces price barriers for those covered by insurance. It may also affect the supply side or the payment mechanisms and the incentives under which providers are paid, as well the regulations under which they operate.

The need for change to improve existing health systems and to adjust to new circumstances has resulted in countries in the region from all economic strata seeking health reform. This has been magnified by the dramatic economic gains and rapid growth of the private health sector experienced in recent years in much of Asia.

1.2   CONFERENCE THEMES

In 1994, the Asian Development Bank (ADB), a regional multilateral development bank, identified a lack of documentation of country experience and of dialogue among policy-makers in the public and private sectors within Asia on the growth of the private health sector. In this absence of information and dialogue, some of the basic questions asked were:

- What should the roles of the public and private sectors be in providing and financing health services?
- How can the objectives of the for-profit private sector be expanded to include national health objectives?

- What should the degree of control and regulation of the private sector be with regard to the quality and pricing of services?
- What payment mechanisms are most appropriate for different levels of the health system?
- What are the effects of different payment mechanisms on private and public sector behavior?
- What is the most appropriate role of government in facilitating private sector provision of health care while mitigating its adverse consequences?
- What are the impacts of a growing private health sector on equity and national development?

To address these issues, the ADB sought a mechanism to increase the documentation of and dialogue about changing patterns of health sector financing and provision. As a result, the ADB sponsored the Second Regional Conference on Health Sector Reform: Issues Related to Private Sector Growth. The ADB contracted with the Health Financing Program of Management Sciences for Health to develop the technical content of the conference, commission the papers and manage the regional conference. This conference, held at the Bank in Manila in March 1996, provided a forum for policy discussion by government officials and private sector representatives on how to achieve the benefits of private participation in the health sector while minimizing the risks of negative consequences of that participation.

From these objectives and the questions related to private sector growth, three basic themes were identified for the conference:

- *Financing options and demand-side issues*, including types of public and private financing, health insurance and its effect on costs and demand for health services, willingness to pay for health care, and allocation of health resources
- *Payment mechanisms and supply-side issues*, including regulatory mechanisms, effects of payment mechanisms on provider behavior, supplier-induced demand, and protection of consumers
- *Quality of care issues*, including the measurement of quality, differentials in quality between the public and private sectors, the relationship of costs to quality, the relationship between quality and health outcomes, and the regulation of quality.

1.3   DEMAND-SIDE, SUPPLY-SIDE, AND QUALITY OF CARE ISSUES

This book is addressed to policy-makers and decision-makers in the public and private health sectors. Its objective is not to prescribe actions to take. While the overall set of options available to policy-makers can be identified, each country is unique — with its own history, internal priorities, available resources and political ideology, as well as its singular interaction with the rest of the world. What is an effective strategy in one country may not be appropriate or feasible in another. The challenge to policy research is not to identify what works but rather to understand the conditions that make a policy effective in some settings but not in others. Policy analysis needs to be directed at understanding the factors that create the current experience in a specific setting. It must also identify those areas that can be affected by public intervention in ways that can improve the impact of the health sector. Central to this process is learning from experience and using those lessons to improve future policies. It is hoped that this book will contribute to that process.

This collection of papers is organized into five sections. The first three chapters provide an overview of private health sector growth, public policy, and the major issues related to the macroeconomic conditions, political environment and health situation of countries. An example of the political process facilitating private sector growth in one country is presented. Part II provides a description and analysis of private health sector growth demand-side issues, as well as the experiences of two countries in the region. The supply-side issues of private health sector growth and case studies from two countries are presented in the third section. The fourth deals with quality issues and how they are defined in the context of health reform, with an example from one country. The final section presents conclusions and recommendations based on the preceding chapters.

1.3.1 Overview of private health sector growth issues

An overview of health sector reform issues is given by Rosenthal and Newbrander. They contend that much of the growth accomplished by countries in the region has been driven by the private sector. In view of the expansion of private sector activities in the economy generally, the issue is how much of the social burden of health service delivery and financing can be assigned to the private sector in order to achieve national health goals. They believe that the challenge of health policy research and information sharing is not to learn what works, but rather to try to understand the conditions that make a policy effective in some settings and not in others. They call for greater collaboration between the public and private sectors in planning. According to Rosenthal and Newbrander, the most important policies are those that will lead to greater public sector efficiency, increased financial responsibility on the part of users, more appropriate fee and payment mechanisms, expanded insurance and other financing options, and incentive systems for quality assurance. In some countries, this may require the development of new institutions, new institutional relationships, and new laws or the revision of existing laws and regulations.

Dung describes the political process to increase the private health sector's role through policy reform as it has evolved in Vietnam. He gives an overview of private sector growth in Vietnam, which has been characterized by an extreme increase in small clinics and pharmacies and a lack of hospitals. Facilities are concentrated in urban areas and in the southern provinces. Dung describes the four phases of private health sector growth and some of the problems associated with this growth. The government is developing a policy evaluation model that evaluates processes, context, implementation, and impact. The objectives of government policy are to develop the private health sector further, to concentrate public health resources on providing care for the poor, to develop traditional medicine, and to promote revenue generation in public hospitals to reduce "hidden costs".

1.3.2   Demand-side issues of private health sector growth

As desire for health care services is effectively transformed into demand through various financing mechanisms, policy-makers must deal with a range of issues. An overview of financing issues in health sector reform is provided by Jeffers. He underscores that health financing is not a goal in and of itself but rather a means to the end of mobilizing a volume of resources sufficient to meet the health goals of a country. Although both the public and private sectors appear to be largely supplier driven in the sense that major decisions are made by providers, not consumers, financing, spending and demand have the greatest degree of leverage on the final allocation of resources. He presents some of the significant trends, including the questions being raised in many countries about what to do with public health service delivery systems. Many countries are thinking about privatizing them, and others are raising user fees and charges at public facilities, while private health insurance coverage is currently small but expanding. Jeffers also discusses the positive and negative aspects of national health insurance.

The issues and problems surrounding the expansion of private health services in Korea are reviewed by Yang. With the expansion of national health insurance, some policy-makers have been advocating the stimulation of the private medical sector as a way of improving quality, technology and efficiency in health service delivery. The Korean experience, however, suggests that there are a number of adverse consequences accompanying private medical expansion fueled by rapid expansion of a national health insurance program. Yang reviews some of the problems with overreliance on for-profit providers, including increased and unnecessary demand for services, increased reliance on high-technology equipment, induced demand for expensive services, and higher prices for health services. He offers alternatives to the actual causes of these unintended consequences of the expanded private sector.

The experience in Thailand with private sector expansion and the development of numerous insurance schemes is presented by Mongkolsmai. She describes various social and private insurance schemes to finance health services and gives the reader an overview of the situation in this country. Statistical trends in the growth of private sector facilities and resources are provided. Mongkolsmai concludes by expressing some concerns about quality, equity, increased costs and expanding expenditures.

1.3.3   Supply-side issues of private health sector growth

In Chapter 7, Berman focuses on health provider payment mechanisms and regulatory issues. By using the experience of developed countries, Berman outlines ways in which developing countries could respond to problems accompanying rapid private sector growth. He presents five options for government intervention on the supply side: direct provision of health services; direct financing of private providers; fiscal actions involving taxes, duties on equipment, and providing investment subsidies; regulation and licensing; and provision of information to users, providers and payers. Berman then discusses the major provider payment options (fee-for-service, capitation, case-based payment, budgetary transfer and salary-based payment) and their impact on the cost, effectiveness and quality of services rendered. He concludes with a review of country experiences in the region with payment mechanisms and regulation.

This chapter is followed by the studies of Bhat and Herrin on India and the Philippines, respectively. Bhat analyzes the repercussions of the Indian government's effort to regulate private health sector activities. He focuses on three laws: the Consumer Protection Act, the Medical Council of India and State Medical Council Acts, and the Nursing Home Act. His analysis illustrates how the growth of the private sector has necessitated the government taking on additional powers to regulate the private health sector in the interests of consumers and maintaining professional, licensure and certification standards.

Herrin describes the effects of Philippine government initiatives on private sector growth over several decades. In the Philippines, the private sector has been seen as a prime mover of development. The government, however, continues to play a significant role in the health sector not only as a provider and financier but also as a regulator of health service delivery activities. Herrin demonstrates that the development of the private medical sector in the Philippines has been strongly influenced by the performance of the economy. He recognizes that government policies have shaped and stimulated this growth by encouraging the production of health human resources, providing special financing for private hospital construction, mandating employers to provide health insurance for employees, and initiating health insurance.

1.3.4 Quality of care issues of private health sector growth

Newbrander and Rosenthal provide an overview of quality issues in Chapter 10. They address the difficult question of the definition of quality and the commonly accepted framework for assessing quality: structure, process, outcomes. Various dimensions of quality are presented in the context of health sector reform. Methods for improving quality are reviewed, including the most common forms of licensure and certification. The authors analyze studies that show that the nonprofit sector generally offers higher-quality health service than the public sector but that no such definitive statements can be made about the for-profit private and public sectors. They conclude by identifying ways in which the public and private sectors can collaborate to improve the quality of health care.

Gani describes private sector development in Indonesia and the initiatives introduced in 1981 to encourage public hospitals to operate on a more business-oriented, self-sufficient basis. Public hospitals were given more flexibility and autonomy to operate like private providers by adjusting prices according to market demand and by retaining and utilizing their revenues. Facilities thus have more resources to increase the quality and quantity of services. The initial conversion of five public hospitals into Unit Swadana ("self-sufficient") hospitals has had a great impact on the development of the private sector in the provision and financing of health services. In general, the growing number of Unit Swadana hospitals has made the market for hospital services more competitive. Based on documented reports and observations made in two Unit Swadana hospitals, the concept has been successful in increasing hospital revenue substantially. With additional revenues and flexibility in their utilization, Unit Swadana hospitals have also succeeded in improving the quality of health services.

It should be noted that the three basic themes of the conference are interrelated and the issues discussed in the various chapters overlap. For instance, Gani's chapter touches on both demand- and supply-side issues. However, the Unit Swadana hospitals are presented here as a compelling illustration of how revenue retention can be used to improve the quality of services in public sector facilities.

1.3.5   Conclusion

Chapter 12 reviews the concepts, lessons learned, and implications from the sharing of these experiences on the growth of the private health sector in Asia. This review permits the anchoring of private sector issues in the context of health sector reform and the comparison of different national experiences with translating concerns into action. The chapter recommends further analysis and implementation of the lessons on various levels — national, regional and global.

REFERENCES

Akin, J., Birdsall, N., de Ferranti, D. (1987). *Financing Health Services in Developing Countries: An Agenda for Reform.* Washington, DC: World Bank.

Griffin, C. (1992). *Health Care in Asia: A Comparative Study of Cost and Financing.* Washington, DC: World Bank.

Newbrander, W., Parker, D. (1992). The public and private sectors in health: economic issues. *Int. J. Hlth Planning and Management,* **7** (1), 37–49.

Organization for Economic Cooperation and Development (OECD). (1990). *Health Care Systems in Transition.* Paris: OECD.

World Health Organization (WHO). (1991). *The Public/Private Mix in National Health Systems and the Role of Ministries of Health.* Report of a meeting held in Mexico, July 20–26, 1991. Geneva: WHO, Division of Strengthening of Health Services.

2

Public Policy and Private Sector Provision of Health Services

GERALD ROSENTHAL

Health Economist, Management Sciences for Health

and

WILLIAM NEWBRANDER

Health Economist, Management Sciences for Health

2.1 INTRODUCTION

This chapter provides an overview of issues related to public/private sector interaction in the provision of health services. It considers first the general development context within which these issues will be addressed, and explores some of the implications of this broader context for national health care priorities and policies. It then presents some of the conceptual arguments for public intervention in the production and distribution of health services. It explores the range of policy options currently being implemented as part of health care reform efforts; in particular, those related to expansion of access and public sector resource limits. It considers actual and potential roles for private provision of services within these policy options and suggests directions for policies that can reinforce the potential synergy of public and private efforts to improve the effectiveness of health services.

2.1.1 Regional economic development and private sector expansion

Any discussion of sectoral policies in Asia needs to begin with a recognition that economic growth is the overriding public priority for most of the countries in the region. For many, it has been a successful quest, producing annual rates of per capita growth from 1980 to 1993 that are greater than 3 per cent for some countries and over twice that for the most successful (see Table 2.1). Even without China and India, countries where per capita GNP increased at a rate over 3 per cent per year

Private Health Sector Growth in Asia: Issues and Implications. Edited by W. Newbrander.
© 1997 John Wiley & Sons, Ltd.

represented more than 520 million people. For many of these people, economic
growth has meant increasing incomes, improvements in consumption, and reduced
economic vulnerability. The positive achievements in the region have reinforced the
political and social consensus that has accounted for this consistent economic
performance.

Much of this economic growth has been driven by private sector expansion. The
private sector has provided the greatest share of investment and capital expansion,
opened new domestic and international markets, and generated employment. Public
policies have been adopted to facilitate access to capital, provide tax incentives for
investment, ease restrictions on imports and exports, and permit companies a wide
range of operational latitude in their organization and operations. For some countries,
economic growth has also meant modifying long-standing policies of domestic
protection and restrictions on foreign investment and ownership of productive
capacity. It is within this setting that health policy issues are being addressed.

2.1.2   Health sector priorities and national policies

The centrality of private sector production of goods and services in national
development strategies creates the context for the present discussion. The public
commitment to encourage and support private sector expansion will also be reflected
in health policies. For instance, the policies to expand private services in Vietnam
and the National Health Insurance program in Korea both reflect extensions of

Table 2.1. Central Government Expenditure for Health in Selected Asian Countries.

| Country | Growth rate, 1980–93 | | Government expenditure as percentage of GDP, 1993 | Health as percentage of government expenditure | |
	GDP per capita	Government consumption		1980	1993
India	3.0	6.2	11.0	1.6	1.9
China	NA	10.8	9.0	NA	0.4
Nepal	2.0	NA	9.0	3.9	4.7
Bangladesh	2.1	NA	14.0	6.4	NA
Mongolia	0.2	NA	18.0	NA	NA
Pakistan	3.1	8.0	14.0	NA	NA
Sri Lanka	2.7	5.6	9.0	4.9	5.2
Indonesia	4.2	4.8	10.0	2.5	2.7
Philippines	−0.6	1.0	9.0	4.3	3.0
Papua New Guinea	0.6	0.6	21.0	8.6	7.9
Thailand	6.4	4.6	10.0	4.1	8.2
Malaysia	3.5	3.9	13.0	5.1	5.7
Korea	8.2	6.1	11.0	1.2	1.0
Hong Kong	5.4	5.7	9.0	NA	NA
Singapore	6.1	6.3	9.0	7.0	6.1

Note: NA, not applicable.
Source: World Bank (1995).

national policies rather than unique responses to sectoral issues (see Chapters 3 and 5). Yet, simply applying national policies for economic development to health may fail to recognize the special characteristics of the sector or to address the strategic priorities that public health policies need to address.

One traditional role of government is to support general health and welfare. For most countries, this includes efforts to facilitate access to needed health services as well as to assure their quality and distribution. Yet, while assuring the health of its citizens is a priority for virtually all countries, efforts to move toward this goal draw on common resources and are affected by the rules influencing all public activities. Commitment of resources and priorities for health must be balanced with other, equally compelling, national priorities in the context of overall economic development.

The issue to be addressed is rarely whether there should be private provision of health services. For most countries throughout the world, private providers account for a significant share of services utilized and private expenditures provide many of the resources. Within Asia in 1990, none of the 14 countries for which data were available reported less than 20 per cent of total health expenditures from private sources (see Table 2.2). For 10 of the 14, the private share was greater than 50 per cent and for three countries — India, Hong Kong, and Thailand — the private share exceeded 75 per cent (World Bank, 1993). In terms of the share of GNP, private expenditure for health care in these countries ranged from less than 1.0 per cent to 4.7 per cent, indicating a significant level of private economic activity within the sector, as well as considerable variation among countries.

There is an underlying perspective to the observations made here. Policy-making is conceptualized as a process of specific interventions or "changes in the rules" designed

Table 2.2. Distribution of Public and Private Expenditure for Health in Selected Asian Countries, 1990.

Country	Total	Percentage of GNP		Relative share (%)	
		Public	Private	Public	Private
India	6.0	1.3	4.7	21.7	78.3
China	3.5	2.1	1.4	60.0	40.0
Nepal	4.5	2.2	2.3	48.9	51.1
Bangladesh	3.2	1.4	1.8	43.7	56.3
Laos	2.5	1.0	1.5	40.0	60.0
Sri Lanka	3.7	1.8	1.9	48.6	51.4
Indonesia	2.0	0.7	1.3	35.0	65.0
Philippines	2.0	1.0	1.0	50.0	50.0
Papua New Guinea	4.4	2.8	1.6	63.6	36.4
Thailand	5.0	1.1	3.9	22.0	78.0
Malaysia	3.0	1.3	1.7	43.3	56.7
Korea	6.6	2.7	3.9	40.9	59.1
Hong Kong	5.7	1.1	4.6	19.3	80.7
Singapore	1.9	1.1	0.8	57.9	42.1

Source: World Bank (1993).

to affect the activities and outcomes of the health sector (Rosenthal, 1970). Effective policy-making is essentially pragmatic, seeking to understand how the current system works and why it works that way. From this assessment, actions that might improve performance can be identified and, if desired, implemented. In the case of private sector provision of health services, health policy-makers need to (Newbrander and Parker, 1992):

- Ask how the existing and potential strengths of the private sector can be drawn upon to achieve public health priorities
- Identify actions to take to ensure that expanded private production of health services does not come at the expense of public priorities.

While we may assess the theoretical impact of a given policy, the actual outcome depends on other factors within the sector, including other policies. New policies affect the already changing performance of the health sector. There are other policy-makers, with other priorities and interests, whose actions affect the ability of the health sector to meet its public objectives and whose actions limit the policy choices available to improve health sector performance. The commitment to private sector development as a central component of general development policy establishes a context within which health policy must be developed. This means that effective conceptual and operational arguments for treating the health sector differently are crucial.

2.2   ECONOMIC ARGUMENTS FOR PUBLIC INTERVENTION

A focus of this book is on using the private sector more effectively to meet public health goals by identifying policies that can improve the quality, distribution, and cost effectiveness of private production and distribution of health services. This emphasis reflects both operational and strategic realities. Operationally, the private sector is already a major player in the delivery of health services and, increasingly, it is also the major source of new investment. These trends are likely to be supported in most countries in the region by other general development policies. From a strategic perspective, health priorities need to be met within this context.

From a technical perspective, we are interested in the strengths and limitations of market-based allocations in determining the volume and distribution of health services and the economic conditions that argue for public provision, regulation, and subsidy of goods and services. Most observations about the normative impacts of the market are based on the behavior of buyers and sellers in what economists call a perfectly competitive market.[1] In such a market, a large number of buyers interact with a large number of sellers to set prices at a level that will make the amount of goods or services fully informed buyers desire exactly equal to the amount fully informed providers want to supply.

---

[1] Virtually all of the observations made in this discussion could be qualified by a number of conditions and exceptions. However, the dynamic described here is generally consistent with the normative arguments for market-based resource allocation and is intended as background for the following discussion.

The conditions that engender efficient outcomes in a perfectly competitive market are rarely satisfied in reality. The economic basis for public production and subsidy emphasizes public action to compensate for the failure (inability) of the market to provide an efficient allocation of resources (see Chapter 4, as well as Arrow, 1963; de Ferranti, 1984; Griffin, 1989; Akin *et al.*, 1987). Certain characteristics of a market may also result in levels of production that are higher or lower than is socially optimal. In the absence of demonstrated market failure, however, efficiency considerations argue for less, rather than more, public intervention.

Although the basic economic arguments are straightforward, many aspects of the market for health services present challenges for public response that depend more on noneconomic assessments of social and political priorities. Some health services, such as public health and infectious and communicable disease management, are inherently public, since private producers will always produce too few of these services. However, for other important services, particularly acute and curative personal care, the arguments for public provision are less obvious, since the private sector can and does produce a significant proportion of these services in many settings.

In the simplest terms, the desired public/private mix is often assessed as a matter of balancing efficiency and equity considerations. For this perspective, the private sector is typically seen as being more efficient, and the public sector, as more equitable. However, life is rarely this simple. Where countries have chosen to produce and distribute services directly, the challenge is to achieve reasonable levels of efficiency without sacrificing commitment to the goals of equity of distribution and quality of care. This usually leads to policies designed to make public producers and consumers act more like private producers and consumers in order to take advantage of the efficiency of the private market. Where the private sector is the predominant source of services, the public challenge is to capture the efficiency advantages of the private market while paying sufficient attention to equity and quality concerns to meet public performance criteria. This often leads to public policies designed to make private providers act more like public providers and to facilitate entry of public consumers into private markets. In fact, there are few "pure" forms currently operational.

The economic analysis presented here emphasizes the strengths of the market and describes government intervention as being directed only at offsetting market failures to improve efficiency. The traditional economic perspective starts from the view that the market is the appropriate setting for making resource allocation decisions unless market failures require public intervention. In many countries, public production has often been justified on the grounds that private markets would not provide the desired level of access to services, particularly for rural populations, where the markets are too small to generate competitive economic returns, and for poor populations, where the capacity for economic participation is too limited. In some cases, however, the priority of public production has also reflected ideological considerations, as in Vietnam prior to its recent shift to market socialism. In many developing countries, the situation reflects the inheritance of public services established under colonial rule, which are sustained by the political and economic necessity of maintaining high levels of public employment and the political importance of the population it serves.

2.3   PUBLIC/PRIVATE POLICY INTERACTIONS

In Asia, health policy initiatives reflect a growing awareness of the role played by the private sector in meeting the demand for health services and the importance of private resources in paying for services.[2] The interaction between the private and the public sectors is not a new phenomenon in health. However, specific recognition of the role of private providers has been absent from much health planning until recently. Even less attention has been given in the past to the deliberate implementation of policies that expand the capacity of the private sector to contribute to public health objectives (Roth, 1987). The growing need for policies that incorporate private sector investment and production reflects both the political changes that permit more overt private sector responsibility for public priorities and the economic changes that place increasing demands on public resources available for health (Newbrander and Parker, 1992).

The increased policy emphasis on private production implies a shift of operational priorities within the public health sector. One objective is the ability to direct more public resources to prevention and health promotion, activities for which the private market is often less effective. A growing private capacity to deal with needed curative services provides the opportunity to achieve this objective. However, responding to the opportunity will require significant changes in current methods of planning and resource allocation within the public sector. Implementing such changes requires both political commitment and managerial capacity.

Private production of services involves risks as well as opportunities. The economic characteristics of the health care market and the growing levels of demand can combine to divert resources from effective services and toward provider revenue generation. If the public sector role as producer of services is to shrink, its role as market regulator and quality assurer will inevitably have to expand. These activities also require resources. The experience of having good laws and inadequate monitoring and enforcement capacity is widespread in Asia and elsewhere. The structure of the health industry, with large numbers of formal and informal providers, diverse distribution, and low capital investment coupled with generally poor public records and registration, makes the regulatory role both difficult and expensive.

2.3.1   Which public priorities?

In addressing its health priorities, each country starts from a unique strategic position. Yet all countries, regardless of the structure and organization of their health services, face increasing pressures on public resources to address problems of illness and to support the provision of health services. For the most well-developed countries, these pressures come primarily from the combination of new technologies and new disease patterns reflected in longer life and increasing chronic disease. In the

---

[2]For the purposes of this discussion, the private sector refers to all nongovernmental producers and financiers of services and includes not-for-profit as well as profit-oriented organizations. For a more detailed discussion of issues related to this definition, see Berman and Rannan-Eliya (1993).

least-developed countries, the same pressures are present but are exacerbated by high rates of population growth and dependence on the public sector for providing acute care as well as preventive and primary health services.

Overcoming resource constraints is not a goal of policy, but a necessary condition for implementing health policies directed at improving health status, ensuring quality of care, extending access to services, and protecting consumers. The test of strategies to deal with resource limitations needs to focus on their effects on these public health objectives. The following discussion explores two lines of initiatives of growing importance in implementing health sector reform: improving public sector efficiency; and, shifting more financial responsibility for personal health services to the user. Each of these policy areas are stimulated by limitations of public sector health resources, but the effectiveness of the policies depends on private sector responses. Moreover, each has implications for the critical goals related to quality, access, and consumer protection.

2.3.2   Policies to improve public sector efficiency

In every country, a significant share of the public resources devoted to health is used for the production and distribution of health services. This is as true when the public share is small as when it is large. In the long run, no real increase in public sector efficiency can be achieved unless the operating focus is on performance and outcomes and the costs of producing them (Mills, 1995). In fact, almost all of the current operating information on public providers focuses on the inputs rather than the outputs. Where output measures are used, they tend to be aggregate (e.g., number of patients or surgical procedures). Although such information tells us how much is being used and what it is being used for in the aggregate, little information is available that tells us what is produced with it. Similarly, a greater emphasis on performance will have no impact if managers in the system have little ability to influence the way resources are used.

In many public systems, only the fees generated from users are under the direct management of the institution. To the extent that the financing alternatives being considered will generate more resources directly at the institutional level, more flexibility is essential. This development will provide increased opportunities for performance-related incentives and require more creative options for assuring that the incentives support the overall efficiency and effectiveness of the institution, not just the service or the staff with the revenue generation opportunity. Further, to support real efficiency, the reward structure of the system must reflect the levels of performance achieved. In fact, many of the current incentives for individuals and organizations related to items such as salaries and budget levels are established in ways that permit little modification in response to performance. Although no simple solutions are available to provide the means for linking rewards to performance, it is important to emphasize that the absence of incentives related to performance greatly limits the ability to achieve efficient levels of production.

Perhaps more essential in the long run are efforts to modify the mix of public services demanded by the population to emphasize services that are likely to have the greatest long-term impact on mortality and morbidity. In economic terms, these are efforts to improve the allocative efficiency of public expenditures through improved budgeting on the resource side and more effective referral systems on the service delivery side. In most settings, improvements in allocative efficiency would be reflected in shifts of resources from treatment to prevention for selected illnesses (e.g., infant diarrhea and vaccine-preventable diseases). A more difficult shift is from more intensive late care to less intensive early care (World Bank, 1993). The shift to less intensive care would include more effective use of community-based health centers and posts and a general shift away from specialty and intensive care institutional settings.

Many factors make the achievement of improved resource allocation within public service provision difficult. Even when the intention is clear, resource constraints and the political nature of the budgetary process often limit the ability of less intensive service providing units to deliver simple basic services. In most public systems, resource constraints fall most heavily on nonhospital activities. Hospital services incorporate most of the skilled personnel, tend to be concentrated in urban areas, and provide services to public employees and other politically consequential constituencies. The resulting absence of drugs, unavailability of trained staff, and limited hours of service in many public primary care settings all serve to demonstrate to users of services that self-referral to other institutional settings is a more effective way to use services. As a result, demand either is shifted to more intensive public service delivery settings, is shifted to the private sector, or remains unsatisfied (Mulou et al., 1992).

Moves toward allocative efficiency are significantly reinforced when policies incorporate efforts to strengthen the capacity of the private sector to deliver acute curative services and to improve access to private services for those currently dependent on public services. However, the limits of publicly provided services already produce a significant demand for private services. Studies of utilization based on household surveys have demonstrated that many users of public services also buy drugs and supplies from the private sector, frequently as part of the same episode of treatment (Akin et al., 1985; Gwynne and Zschock, 1989). Providing a prescription for patients when there are no drug supplies in the clinics is a direct recognition of the private sector's role in providing services to patients of the public system. Some individuals also choose to be treated by private providers for reasons of greater access, hours of service that permit receipt of services without lost wages, and the expectation of higher quality care. The choices may also reflect the nature of the health problem, anticipated costs for services, and timing, but such behavior is found in families at all economic levels.

Increasing the scale and effectiveness of the role of private providers in meeting health care demand typically requires government action. The range of policy options available depends significantly on the potential size of the private market. This reflects both the population and the existence of financing policies that facilitate private demand. For many countries in Asia, the potential volume of demand has demonstrated the ability to attract the needed capital from international as well as domestic sources. The attraction of such markets already provides opportunities for more creative public/private relationships, such as low-income service delivery set-asides for new private construction in India.

On the stimulative side, private providers need legal standing to gain access to investment and credit and to the financial institutions that can provide it. Tax and import concessions can be used to affect the scale and distribution of private providers by targeting lower costs of production to areas of high public priority. On the restrictive side, expansion of private provision of services may be supported contingent on meeting specific equipment and procedural requirements or, in some cases, specific public service delivery requirements (e.g., requirement that a facility that provides emergency services be licensed as a hospital). Many of these policies have been incorporated into the general economic development strategy in Asia and already contribute to the growth of private sector provision of health services.

2.3.3   Policies to increase users' financial responsibility

Opportunities exist for reducing the demand for public services and increasing the efficiency with which public resources are used, as noted above. However, most countries are also exploring the potential for expanding increasing user fees for acute curative care. In countries where the public sector is the major producer, the net effect of this change is to make more public resources available for noncurative public health services. Where a large proportion of the care is provided in the private sector, such strategies are intended both to reduce demand for public services and to generate revenues.

Three sources are available for increasing revenues for public health services: (1) increasing taxes or the public health share of existing taxes; (2) generating revenues from users of services; and, (3) expansion of external cooperation. Contemporary realities have directed much evolving policy toward revenue generation from users since national budgets are already hard pressed and donors have increasingly emphasized sustainability (that is, requiring that recipient countries meet the recurrent costs of activities developed with external assistance). Further, appropriately implemented policies to generate revenues from users will also contribute to the efficiency of the system by linking demand to the actual costs of providing the services.

Many different options exist for obtaining increased revenues from users. In addition to direct fees, insurance strategies whose premiums are based on wages or other links to the ability to pay offer opportunities for combining user revenues with risk pooling. These options are not mutually exclusive, and the policy development process needs to consider all of them separately and in combination. Each strategy for public sector revenue generation also modifies the context for private production of services.

2.3.3.1 Direct fees.   In almost every developing country, efforts are underway to assess, implement, or expand the generation of revenues from the users of public services. This activity reflects not only the need for revenues but also a growing awareness that the resource limitations in the system already impose direct costs on the users. Although the goal of service without cost remains in principle, in practice users are increasingly bearing some of the costs of publicly provided services. In many countries, shortages of supplies and drugs are dealt with by effectively imposing the responsibility for buying these items on the user. Giving a patient a prescription in place of the medicine is, in effect, making the patient responsible for payment in order to receive treatment.

This reality conflicts with the equity principles that should guide the distribution of public resources. The imposition of charges on the users in this manner is not related systematically to the relative ability of the patient to afford them. Rather, it reflects the providers' inability to treat the patient due to limits of budget and logistics. This often means that no one pays in the early part of the fiscal year, whereas everyone has to pay toward the end of the year when there are no supplies. Given such problems, governments increasingly recognize that formal cost-recovery strategies with clear criteria for waivers and exemptions can be designed that will both generate revenues and be far more equitable in their impacts.

The prices paid by users of drugs and supplies in the private sector are usually considerably higher than the costs for the same commodities in the public system.[3] It is clear that the relatively high use of private providers by people of all economic levels in most countries indicates qualitative differences perceived by users, not just lack of resources. The imposition of user fees will accentuate these differences by changing the relative prices. At the same time, retention of revenues at the provider level and the ability to manage these resources according to institutional needs represents an opportunity to improve the competitive performance of public institutions.

The move toward expanded cost recovery in public systems also equalizes exposure to the financial risks associated with the use of health services. It needs to be emphasized that many of the current expenditures that people make are to compensate for quality deficiencies in the public sector services. Most important is the absence of drugs and other supplies, followed typically by poor service standards. Implementing a cost-recovery program without demonstrating significant improvements in these attributes will not yield satisfactory results. People have demonstrated a willingness, reflected in the growth of the private sector, to incur charges for better services. Not all of the users of private services are well-to-do or insured. Many are individuals who are willing to incur much higher monetary costs to get timely and adequate attention.

Demand responds to changes in the relative price of public services. The objective of the fee waiver or exemption system is to protect access for the poor and minimize the number of patients who turn to self-care, or no care, in response to the new costs. Where private providers are available, there is likely to be some shift from public provision to private provision (Alderman and Gertler, 1989). The equity implications of a reduction in public demand resulting from imposition of user fees cannot be determined without knowing more about demand in the market as a whole. Nevertheless, it is important to monitor the client mix and assess in an ongoing process the impact of the cost-recovery effort on the distribution and use of services.

---

[3]In many countries with cost recovery, the revenues generated are used to offset inadequate budgets for drugs and supplies. Such purchases are usually made locally at prices many times higher than centrally purchased public supplies, thus reducing the impact of user fees in terms of contribution to output.

2.3.3.2 Expanding insurance options. The move toward user fees as a source of public health financing expands the potential importance of insurance strategies and offers additional options for private sector service provision. When the use of services involves a financial risk for patients, insurance programs can facilitate access by spreading these risks over a greater population and limiting the potential costs of care to individuals. Critical to the expansion of private sector roles in the provision of health services, particularly for inpatient services, is the development of expanded provisions for insurance and other prepayment or savings instruments for a significant part of the population. As a result, policies to encourage the development of expanded insurance options for the population are an important component of most national health financing and revenue generation efforts.

All these revenue-generating activities are interrelated. Where public health services are widespread and essentially free, people have little incentive to pay for them. Instead, they use their personal resources to offset the limitations of the public system by buying medicines not provided by the public system, using private providers for off-hours care, and turning to traditional medicine for more services. In such a setting, the potential of social and private insurance expansion is quite limited. Where charges are levied for services in public as well as private settings, consumers will seek to have a wider range of choices and to protect themselves from the financial uncertainties associated with health service utilization.

Insurance mechanisms can be public or private in any combination, but widespread insurance coverage means that a large part of the population has the ability to pay for services. Insurance also provides an instrument for enhancing the ability to purchase services of lower-income populations by directing subsidies to the demand side of the market. However, the development of provider-based insurance, such as health maintenance organizations, may be limited by the inability to spread the risk over a sufficiently large insured population. Providing services to small employee groups can put a single provider at excessive financial risk by making it impossible to spread the costs of a few expensive illnesses across a large enough group of payers. To facilitate more private participation, consideration should be given to developing reinsurance mechanisms whereby the extreme risks are pooled over all of the providers. Such an initiative would protect all providers from extreme risks and demonstrate the commitment to facilitate broader options for beneficiaries and providers.

Unfortunately, in many developing countries the expansion of insurance options is limited by other deficiencies in infrastructure. The absence of effective financial institutions and risk-pooling instruments limits the supply of insurance options. Collection and management systems and actuarial bases for establishing premiums, identifying relative risk, and establishing cash flow requirements need to be established. On the demand side, lack of experience with credit and prepayment structures may also limit the size of the potential market and place insurers at increased risk.

The expansion of insurance coverage also provides opportunities for subsidizing the consumption of health services through the demand side of the market. The growing interest in the use of demand subsidies is one form of implementing distributive (equity) commitments without losing the efficiency incentive present in a more competitive market. A subsidy is designed to reduce the cost of participation in public or private insurance mechanisms for those able to pay only part or none of the costs. It would allow wider participation in these insurance programs and bring the beneficiaries of public support into the general private market for health care services. By retaining the personal financial responsibility for consuming health services and by giving the beneficiary the right to choose where services are obtained on a competitive basis, such systems have the potential for supporting more efficient production of services and a more effective meeting of consumer demand. The health card program in Thailand incorporates many of these characteristics. In Colombia, more than one million poor people are covered by insurance pools that pay for their health services. Similar programs are being implemented in Chile and other Latin American countries.

2.4   KEY PRIVATE SECTOR ISSUES FOR PUBLIC POLICY-MAKERS

The discussion has identified areas where public sector policies aimed at extending access and redirecting public resources depend on private sector actions. These strategies focus on reducing demand, improving efficiency, and generating increased revenues in the public sector. However, these public sector strategies reinforce an expanded role for private provision of services. In addition to the general commitment of countries in the region to support private sector development as part of overall development strategy, there are reasons for expanding the role of the private market in the provision of health services. These include clearer incentives for efficiency, the ability to acquire capital, and, most important, the potential to redirect limited public resources to public priorities.

To be effective, however, planning for an increased role for the private sector also needs to recognize the limitations of markets for meeting some public goals in health services. It requires a public emphasis on assuring the consistency of private production with public health objectives. Accomplishing these objectives will require attention to a number of issues, including equity, access, efficiency, and effectiveness. (See the glossary for definitions of these terms.)

A recurring central issue is the relatively weak incentive system in the private market for quality assurance. The effectiveness of the market in allocating resources depends, in large measure, on the assumption that both buyers and sellers are able to determine the quality and quantity of the goods and services being exchanged for money. In the health sector, this assumption is only partly met. In terms of physical surroundings and the availability of materials and services, users of the system have considerable ability to assess quality. However, it is fundamental to the nature of medical practice that patients assign to providers the responsibility for determining what should be provided, thereby giving up a role of importance in achieving market efficiency in quality as well as cost minimization. Increasing the role of the market in health care provision therefore increases the need for implementation of more effective, demonstrable quality assurance procedures for private as well as public providers. Although forms of implementation vary, development of consumer protection regulations and clinical and service provision norms may still require public activities and use public resources.

None of the issues noted above are unique to the private sector. Public sector provision faces, and in many countries fails, the same tests of equity, access, and effectiveness. Public policy attention to these issues is equally important regardless of the relative importance of the sectors. However, the form in which these issues need to be addressed will be different as the relative roles shift. The move to increased recognition of private sector roles opens the way for more effective public policy.

The limitations of this process also need to be recognized. No amount of policy analysis and health care financing reform can make a poor country into a rich one. Development of the health sector occurs within, and is limited by, the overall development context. The expansion of private production of services will inevitably increase the resources flowing into the sector but may not increase the resources for the most cost-effective public health priorities. Establishing realistic goals and setting appropriate priorities for the use of public funds is essential (Newbrander and Parker, 1992). Although the allocation of private funds may be guided by different criteria, it draws on a common set of resources and influences the allocation of public resources whether or not planning has considered these effects. By specifically considering these effects, better strategies for the use of public funds can be developed and implemented.

This chapter provides an introduction to the forms that such policies might take. Many principles and strategies designed to improve the generation and management of resources in the health system are described in this book. Although all are important, they do not represent a "magic" solution to the fundamental problems of inadequate resources and high need for services. Rather, they represent opportunities to improve the ability to focus resources on high-priority health activities in the public sector and to make more effective and efficient use of the resources of the private sector for this task. In this sense, realistic expectations are essential. The impacts of successful strategies, in terms of additional revenues and improved use of existing resources, will only evolve gradually.

REFERENCES

Akin, J., Birdsall, N., de Ferranti, D. (1987). *Financing Health Services in Developing Countries: An Agenda for Reform*. Washington, DC: World Bank.

Akin, J., Guilkey, D., Griffin C., Popkin, B. (1985). *The Demand for Primary Health Services in the Third World*. Totowa, NJ: Rowman and Allenheld.

Alderman, H., Gertler, P. (1989). *The Substitutionality of Public and Private Care for the Treatment of Children in Pakistan*. Washington, DC: World Bank.

Arrow, K. (1963). Uncertainty and the welfare economics of medical care. *American Economic Review*, **53**, 941–973.

Berman, P., Rannan-Eliya, R. (1993). *Factors Affecting the Development of Private Health Care Provision in Developing Countries*. Major Applied Research Paper No. 9. Bethesda, MD: Health Financing and Sustainability Project.

de Ferranti, D. (1984). Strategies for paying for health services in developing countries. *World Health Statistics Quarterly*, **37** (4), 428–442.

Griffin, C. (1989). *Strengthening Health Services in Developing Countries through the Private Sector*. IFC Discussion Paper No. 4. Washington, DC: World Bank.

Gwynne, G., Zschock, D. (1989). *Health Care Financing in Latin America and the Caribbean, 1985–89: Findings and Recommendations*. Stony Brook, NY: SUNY-Dept. of Economics.

Mills, A. (1995). *Improving the Efficiency of Public Sector Health Services in Developing Countries: Bureaucratic versus Market Approaches*. London: London School of Tropical Medicine and Hygiene.

Mulou, N., Thomason, J., Edwards, K. (1992). The rise of private practice: a growing disquiet with public services? *Papua New Guinea Medical Journal*, **35**(3), 7–14.

Newbrander, W., Parker, D. (1992). The public and private sectors in health: economic issues. *Int. J. Hlth Planning and Management*, **7**(1), 37–49.

Rosenthal, G. (1970). Planning for health care — the choice of policies. In: Sheldon, A., Baker, F. (Eds). *Systems and Medical Care*. Boston: MIT Press.

Roth, G. (1987). *The Private Provision of Public Services in Developing Countries*. New York: Oxford University Press.

World Bank. (1993). *World Development Report 1993: Investing in Health*. New York: Oxford University Press.

World Bank. (1995). *World Development Report 1995: Workers in an Integrating World*. New York: Oxford University Press.

3

The Political Process to Increase The Private Health Sector's Role in Vietnam

PHAM HUY DUNG

Professor of Epidemiology, Hanoi Medical School, and Vice Director, Center for Social Sciences for Health

3.1 INTRODUCTION

Many changes are occurring in Vietnam. The laws and policies sanctioning the planned and deliberate growth of the private health sector are manifestations of some of these changes. This chapter provides an overview of the current situation of the private health sector in Vietnam. It also presents the legal basis for the development of the private health sector, describes the phases of private sector growth, presents survey data on policy-makers' perceptions of private health sector development, and makes recommendations for appropriate support to private health providers and the improvement of the health system.

The overview describes private health facilities, financing, human resources and utilization and is based on:

- A study of the private health sector in eight Vietnamese provinces in 1992
- A case study of private health sector growth in Ho Chi Minh City from 1993 to 1995
- A rapid appraisal for updating the data on private health sector growth in 53 provinces in 1995.

The remainder of the chapter, dealing with the legal basis and political process to promote private sector growth, is based on Vietnam's health policies, laws, guidelines, and regulations, and the results of interviews with health policy-makers.

3.2 OVERVIEW OF THE PRIVATE HEALTH SECTOR IN VIETNAM

3.2.1 Introduction

The development of private health services in Vietnam has been a natural process of adjustment to growing demand. The experience of Ho Chi Minh City (formerly

Private Health Sector Growth in Asia: Issues and Implications. Edited by W. Newbrander.
© 1997 John Wiley & Sons, Ltd.

Saigon) exemplifies this process. Before 1975, there were many private health services in the city. Private health services were administered by the Ministry of Health (MOH) with the participation of professional societies. After 1975, private health services were merged into the national health system. With the so-called re-education campaign, the city health office saw the need to recognize and regulate the private sector due to the extensive unofficial or illegal private health services and sale of drugs.

In 1979, restrictions were eased as the city health office allowed public physicians to have their own evening consultation rooms in order to supplement their incomes, as well as to respond to pent-up demand. In 1980, in order to develop a mix of public and private pharmacies and to control the black market in drugs, the health office organized the administration of private pharmacies and private health services and integrated it into its own departments. Thus, although the private health sector was not officially sanctioned at the country level, Ho Chi Minh City had moved to solve its own problems in response to market demand by recognizing and regulating it.

In 1989, this phenomenon was extended to the entire country. The MOH issued decrees related to private pharmacies and health services. In implementing these decrees, many provincial and city health offices organized special departments for the administration of nonpublic health and pharmaceutical services.

These decrees were the result of a liberalizing process initiated by the 6th Communist Party Congress in 1986. It eventually led to the adoption by the 7th Communist Party Congress in 1991 of an "open" policy, known as market socialism. At the 4th meeting of the Central Committee, in 1993, a policy of a diversified public and private health service system was adopted. It led to the legalization of informal health providers. Laws concerning private practice by health and pharmaceutical professionals were approved by Parliament and decreed by the state president in October 1993. Then, Cabinet and the MOH issued guidelines and regulations for the implementation of these laws.

Vietnam has experienced slow economic growth: per capita GNP was only US $170 in 1993. The government's health budget in 1994 was US $2.13 per person for the population of 72.5 million. The mix of the health system in Vietnam is predominantly public: of the 678 general hospitals, only two are private. Conversely, 70 per cent of the 7500 clinics and polyclinics in the country are private. These figures mask the fact that the majority of the public polyclinics are large, while the private clinics are small, usually having only a single health provider rendering services. Another area where the private health sector is emerging is the sale of drugs at pharmacies.

Detailed and accurate data on the private health sector — its providers, facilities, services, and utilization patterns — are unavailable at this time. What limited information is available is presented below.

3.2.2 Facilities and services

The classifications of public and private are not applicable to all categories of health provision because Vietnam is in a period of transition. Government health facilities include those under the MOH and other ministries and governmental agencies, as well as those under provincial authorities. Nongovernmental health facilities include health facilities run by individuals, private collectives, the community, or charitable organizations.

Legally, private health services are categorized into three groups: the private practice of medicine; the private practice of traditional medicine; and, the private practice of pharmacists. The private practice of medicine includes hospitals, midwifery services, general or specialized polyclinics, rooms for dentistry and radiology, units for plastic surgery, and rehabilitation, nursing, and family planning services. The private practice of traditional medicine includes hospitals and consultation rooms for traditional medicine, as well as services such as acupuncture, massage, digipuncture, and inhalation. The private practice of pharmacists includes those working in private pharmacies, dealers or commissioned sellers for a pharmaceutical enterprise, private pharmaceutical companies, limited responsibility companies, shareholder companies, and business units of traditional medicine.

Drug production and distribution in Vietnam are now under the administration of the MOH. Pharmaceutical companies and factories are revenue-generating services of the government. Most finished pharmaceuticals are produced in-country. Pharmaceutical materials can be imported for the production of tablets or ampoules. The proportion of imported finished products represents 10 to 30 per cent of the monetary value of the drugs used annually. According to data of the MOH's Department of Health Statistics, the total value of drug products in 1994 was VN $143 891 million (US $1 = VN $11 000).

The number of private services that received official licenses from provincial health authorities is shown in Table 3.1. However, these figures undoubtedly under-report the true size of the private health sector.

3.2.3 Providers

There are two groups of private health sector providers: (1) full-time providers who own private facilities and collect fees directly from their clients; and, (2) part-time private providers who are on the staff of public health facilities but work during the evening or at other times and collect fees directly from their clients. For the time being, there are no trade organizations of private physicians, pharmacists, or traditional practitioners; they are integrated into general societies of all physicians, pharmacists, or traditional practitioners.

The data from a 1992 study on human resources in eight provinces (Ha Giang, Thai Binh, Thanh Hoa, Khanh Hoa, Gia Lai, Tay Ninh, Vinh Long, and Hanoi) reveal the number of providers in seven categories (see Table 3.2). Almost half of the private health providers come from public services (and work part-time in both sectors). Almost all the full-time private health providers are those retired from the public health sector. All of them were trained to work in a national health system; none was trained to work in a mixed public and private health system.

The same study shows that there were 4111 private health providers in these eight provinces. An investigation of 230 communes found 166 private health providers. Only one-third of them were licensed. If this were consistent across all categories,

Table 3.1. Number of Licensed Private Providers by Service Category.

Categories of service	Number
Medicine	
Midwifery	148
Clinic	5344
Dentistry	1080
Laboratory	54
X-ray	55
Echography	20
Plastic surgery	18
Rehabilitation unit	10
Nursing service	1352
Family planning service	28
Hospital	2
Pharmacy	
Drug supplier	3560
Pharmacy	3748
Drug enterprise	70
Drug company	27
Drug trade	598
Traditional medicine	
Clinic	2099
Rehabilitation unit	1
Acupuncture unit	191
Hospital	1

Source: Original data collection by author funded by Asian Development Bank for paper submitted to Management Sciences for Health for ADB Regional Conference. Data collection undertaken in collaboration with the Cabinet of the Ministry of Health, 1995.

it would mean that the real number of private health providers in these eight provinces should be approximately three times 4000, i.e. 12 000.

3.2.4   Utilization

There are no data available on the utilization of private health services. Most of the private facilities have not kept records.

During the study of eight provinces in 1992, estimates were made based on interviews in private clinics. The following information was gathered:

- Frequency of clients, by age and by sex: The largest group of patients seen were children (33 per cent), followed by the elderly (22 per cent), teenagers (15 per cent), and women (26 per cent)
- Frequency of diseases: The most common conditions treated were arthritis (15 per cent), asthenia (11 per cent), and asthma and cough (11 per cent)
- Consultation fee: The fee for one consultation is about VN $2000 (US $0.20).

Table 3.2. Health Personnel in Private Practice by Category and Province.

Province	Physicians FT	Physicians PT	Pharmacists FT	Pharmacists PT	Nurses FT	Nurses PT	Assistant pharmacists FT	Assistant pharmacists PT	Midwives FT	Midwives PT	Technicians FT	Technicians PT	Traditional healers FT	Traditional healers PT	Total FT	Total PT
Ha Giang	9	6	7	10	—	—	—	—	—	—	—	—	—	—	16	16
Thai Binh	65	50	8	15	206	—	224	10	—	—	13	6	3	1	519	82
Thanh Hoa	40	18	30	22	—	—	16	—	—	—	—	—	1	—	87	40
Khanh Hoa	26	101	26	17	43	3	61	—	2	3	1	3	145	—	304	127
Gia Lai	12	73	3	4	—	—	22	10	—	12	—	—	40	4	77	103
Tay Ninh	6	109	6	32	24	53	50	34	7	25	2	6	23	9	118	268
Vinh Long	5	82	15	35	—	—	27	—	—	—	—	—	15	—	62	117
Hanoi	300	636	365	331	95	100	38	—	1	7	—	—	159	2	958	1076
Total	463	1075	460	466	368	156	438	54	10	47	16	15	386	16	2141	1829

FT, Full-time; PT, part-time.
Source: Survey conducted by Center for Human Resources for Health for Ministry of Health and UNICEF, 1993, internal, unpublished paper.

3.2.5   Financing

The financing of health services is diversified. Financing mechanisms include revenue-generating schemes and subsidies. Financing sources include tax-based payments, insurance-based payments, and out-of-pocket payments.

Historically, Vietnam had only public facilities. In the process of transition, public facilities collected fees for services as a means of cost recovery. Thus, some public facilities developed the concept of revenue generation. Facilities were maintained in order to meet the needs of the poor. Nongovernmental facilities include communal health centers financed by collective farms. These facilities became only partially public, being financed partly by the communes' people's committees and partly by the government. Nongovernmental for-profit services consist mainly of private clinics and private pharmacies. Nongovernmental, free-of-charge, and subsidized facilities are those that work under the Red Cross and other nongovernmental organizations.

There are three insurance schemes in Vietnam. The first is the compulsory health insurance for all salaried persons, whether public or private; they must contribute 3 per cent of their salaries to the scheme (1 per cent is paid by the employer and 2 per cent by the employee). The second is the voluntary health insurance being tried in some pilot provinces (including Hai Phong and Hai Hung). The third is a specific private indemnity health insurance (insurance for surgical operations, for example) being developed by the Vietnam Insurance Company (Bao Viet).

3.2.6   Ho Chi Minh City case study

Ho Chi Minh City (formerly Saigon) has had more experience with private health sector providers due to its more developed pre-1975 health and economic system, so it is not surprising that it has the highest number of private health services in Vietnam. This case study includes data on private health sector growth in 1993, 1994, and 1995. While the data from 1993 and 1994 are similar, major changes occurred between 1994 and 1995.

In 1993 in Ho Chi Minh City, there were 2682 individual private clinics, 1416 individual private pharmacies, 33 collective clinics in public hospitals, 22 collective traditional medicine clinics, 300 individual private traditional practitioners, 66 dispensaries with surgical rooms for private surgeons, 17 individual private plastic surgical rooms, 443 private dentists, 17 private midwives, and one private diagnostic center.

The studies showed that there were increases in the number of private consultation rooms and charity clinics in 1994, as well as increases in the number of pharmacies, drug dealers, herbal medicine shops, private drug wholesale shops, and medical representatives. However, there was no significant change in the production and trading of medical equipment and drugs.

3.2.7   Findings

Based on statistics from the MOH's Policy Unit, in 1995 there were 9800 private health providers in the country. They provided mainly primary care. There were a few joint-venture hospitals for tertiary care in Ho Chi Minh City for foreigners and for local people who were able to pay. The development of the private health sector induced the concept and practice of collecting fees in public hospitals.

At present, the private health sector in Vietnam is small and concentrated mainly in urban areas such as Ho Chi Minh City. Table 3.3 shows the regional distribution of private sector facilities and public sector providers in seven regions. Due to historical factors, the private health sector is larger in the south than in the north. However, growth is expected to accelerate faster in the north in the future.

There is now a public policy for private health sector growth. Policy-makers are determined to decentralize, leaving discretionary care to the private sector in order to concentrate public resources on essential care for the poor. Policies for private health sector growth are very cautious, in order to minimize the negative effects while taking advantage of the positive effects. The positive aspects of private sector growth include: complementing and supplementing the services provided by the public sector; reducing per capita state health expenditure on specialty personal health services; making health services and drugs more available; allowing more freedom of choice for consumers for their health services and drugs; and, developing additional health services.

The negative aspects include: the prescribing and selling of unnecessary drugs or interventions; unethical advertisements; provision of unsafe services; the loss of human resources from the public sector; increases in prices of services and drugs; and, the use of public facilities for individual profit.

3.3   THE LEGAL BASIS OF PRIVATE SECTOR DEVELOPMENT

The private health sector can be divided into both formal and informal sectors. The formal private sector consists of licensed private health providers, including

Table 3.3. Private Sector Facilities and Public Health Staff per 100 000 Population in Seven Regions.

Area	Pharmacies	Clinics	Public health staff
Northern Mountain	2	2	196
Red River Delta	5	5	192
Northern Coast	3	3	165
Central Coast	4	5	187
Highland	3	7	228
Eastern Southland	10	20	230
Cuu Long River Delta	2	8	140

Sources: 1. Data on private clinics and pharmacies from original data collection by author funded by Asian Development Bank for paper submitted to Management Sciences for Health for ADB Regional Conference. Data collection undertaken in collaboration with the Cabinet of the Ministry of Health, 1995.
2. Data on public health staff taken from Health Statistic Unit, Ministry of Health, 1995. *Health Statistics in 1994*, Hanoi.
3. Data on regions and population from: National Statistic Department, 1995. *Statistics 1994*, Hanoi.
Note: All facilities and staff figures are per 100 000 population.

traditional practitioners and drug suppliers. Providers in the informal sector do not have licenses. Informal private providers are different from illegal private ones. Informal private providers are informally recognized by the government or local authorities in cases where there are no laws and regulations yet. Illegal private providers are those who do not have licenses when laws and regulations are in effect.

The formal private health sector is quite new in Vietnam. In the former subsidized command economy, there were only state and collective production and distribution channels for health services. Private health services were not permitted. Health care was provided free of charge to every citizen in collective health centers operating together with state hospitals and other state health institutions. Collective health centers were responsible for primary care at the commune level (lowest administrative unit), while state hospitals and other health institutions supplied higher curative and preventive services from the district to central levels.

As mentioned in the introduction, the private health sector started to grow with the adoption of a socialist market-oriented economy. This economic transition started in 1987 with the concept of "mind renewal" (*doi moi tu duy*), a way of rethinking socialist development. The 6th Congress defined this first phase of the transitional period from capitalism to communism, with the main concept being the acceptance of diversified financing, provision, and market mechanisms throughout all sectors.

Based on this shift, the MOH issued the first regulations for private health care providers. However, at that point there were no approved laws for private practice. These laws were introduced only in 1991, after the 7th Communist Party Congress agreed to move from the concept of mind renewal to the practice of "renovation" (*doi moi*). This was the socioeconomic reform that reconfirmed the division of providers into five categories: state, collective, individual, private, and household.

The adoption of open policies paved the way for foreign investment. In January 1993, the Central Committee (elected by the 7th Communist Party Congress) reconsidered health policies at its 4th meeting. The diversification of health care provision and financing was officially recognized.

As a result of these national policies, various laws, guidelines, and regulations were issued regarding the private health sector. These included laws for the private practice of health professionals, pharmacists and traditional practitioners, guidelines for foreign investment in for-profit or not-for-profit health services, and the issuance of licenses for private health sector providers and facilities.

These policies are too new to be judged on the criteria of quality, efficiency, and equity of health care. However, an attempt will be made to examine the strengths and weaknesses of these policies and to recommend policy adjustments to support appropriate private sector growth.

3.4   THE PROCESS OF PRIVATE SECTOR DEVELOPMENT

The process of private health sector growth in Vietnam has consisted of four phases: (1) the development phase; (2) the sensitization phase; (3) the organizational phase; and, (4) the functional phase.

3.4.1   Development phase

Policies for private health sector growth originated from community demand, as well as from the policy orientation of the Party. The origins of community demand for private health services go back to 1975. Before 1975, there were no private services in the Democratic Republic of Vietnam, since health services at all levels were provided by the public sector and community income was relatively low. In 1975, the Democratic Republic of Vietnam became the Socialist Republic of Vietnam. There were large income differences between the populations of the southern and northern provinces. Health demands were not the same among the rich and the poor. While the policy of free health services in the northern provinces was applied to the entire country, private health providers continued to serve those who were willing and able to pay.

At that time, there were no laws, regulations, or guidelines for the private provision of health services. Local authorities considered private practitioners the same as individuals producing handicrafts. Almost all private health providers worked informally at home. Many were staff members of public institutions receiving clients before or after working hours. Private drug sellers sold drugs on the black market.

The concept of market socialism was adopted after assessing past mistakes and shortcomings. In retrospect, the Five-Year Plan of 1976–80 was much too optimistic. It expected modern industry and agriculture to develop throughout the country within a short period based on a centralized command economy. The objectives of this plan were never fully implemented. The annual gross domestic product increase during this period was only 0.4 per cent, though it was intended to be 10 times higher. In 1985, the country was integrated into a subsidized, centrally planned economy. This resulted in low productivity, inflation, and lack of economic progress. By autumn 1985, Vietnam had to adjust to solve the economic crisis.

The process of renovation was gradually formed in the decisions of the Party by means of formal and informal documents, as well as in the resolutions of the National Assembly. The most important decision was to carry out a comprehensive program to shift to a market economy regulated by the state. From 1989 to 1992, the reform declared war on inflation, adopted a new banking system, developed financial policies, used various price-based solutions, enhanced industrial production, promoted foreign investment, encouraged the growth of the private sector, and began rebuilding the country's infrastructure. The reform involved new policies for credit and money, finance and tax, production and administration.

3.4.2   Sensitization phase

In the sensitization phase, the MOH planned the implementation of state laws and government decrees for the private health and pharmaceutical professions proposed by the Cabinet of the Minister of Health. In 1994, the MOH held three regional meetings to discuss the new directions outlined by new laws on private providers. Following this, 53 meetings were organized at the provincial level with the participation of health managers from provincial health offices, provincial health institutions, and district health centers. Their objectives were to acquire knowledge about the criteria and conditions for the private practice of health and pharmaceutical professionals, to get information on the formalities for requesting licenses and levels of authorities delivering licenses, and to develop structures and functions for management mechanisms for private health and pharmaceutical services.

3.4.3   Organizational phase

At the central level, the MOH is responsible for overseeing private health and pharmaceutical professionals and traditional practitioners. The responsible MOH units are the Department of Curative Care, the Department of Pharmacy, and the Department of Traditional Medicine; each department is responsible for administering the private practice of its respective providers. The Cabinet of the Minister is responsible for tracking, reporting on, and evaluating the private practice of health and pharmaceutical professionals.

Licenses for private hospitals and pharmaceutical companies or factories are issued by the MOH and its various advisory boards. Licenses for other private units, such as clinics and dispensaries, are issued by provincial health services. At the provincial level, each provincial health office has a unit for overseeing the private health and pharmaceutical professionals and traditional practitioners.

3.4.4   Functional phase

During the fourth quarter of 1994, the MOH and various provincial health services re-examined private units of medical, traditional medicine, and pharmaceutical services that had obtained licenses under the 1989 MOH regulations. Rural and urban commune people's committees participated in the inspection of private health units to determine which ones were licensed. From 1995 onward, professionals' requests for licenses for private practice were examined quarterly.

A study was conducted in two provinces (Hanoi and Ho Chi Minh City) to evaluate the efficiency, equity, and quality of health care following the implementation of policies on private health practice. The study solicited opinions from MOH administrators and provincial health administrators on how the components of implementation (sensitization and structural and functional organization) could be evaluated.

3.5   POLICY-MAKERS' PERCEPTIONS

To discover the knowledge, attitudes, and practices of key health policy-makers regarding health service efficiency, equity, and quality, in-depth interviews and focus group discussions were held. These issues were reviewed in light of the policy-makers' political orientation and laws, regulations, and guidelines for private health sector growth.

The interviews and focus group discussions were based on these questions:

- What policies were developed to promote private sector growth?
- Why were policies related to health sector growth developed?
- What are the problems or policy issues related to private health sector growth?
- What results are expected from the policy?
- What are the mechanisms and processes for their development?
- How were the policies implemented?

3.5.1 Policies

Several important policies made the birth and growth of the private health sector possible. First, as shown above, policy on private health practice paved the way for the introduction of laws, regulations, and guidelines. Second, service fees in public health services were decreed. Third, the policy on private health practice stimulated the introduction of various health insurance schemes, and three were developed (see section 3.2.5).

The policy on private health practice required the reorganization of health services from the central to the commune level. A number of changes have occurred, including the following:

- The government now contributes more to the network of communal health stations (or health centers). Previously, the ones in rural agricultural regions were financed by collective farms. There were often great variations in compensation for staff, so the government decided to provide salaries for three health workers in each commune
- District hospitals and district health bureaus were integrated into district health centers, and hospital beds are distributed according to population size rather than administrative areas.

3.5.2 Perceptions

There were three phases in the development of policies for private health sector growth: the political orientation phase, the legislative phase, and the executive phase. To understand these, the author developed a model for analysis. Interviews with policy-makers were used to provide insights for the analysis. Four different elements of this sequence were analysed: the policy-making process, the policy context, policy implementation, and policy impact.

Using this policy evaluation model, it was observed that the efficiency, equity, and quality scores of the policy-making process are higher than those of the policy context; those of the policy context are higher than those of policy implementation; and those of policy implementation are higher than those of policy impact.

The key question is why the policy value according to these criteria decreases, from process to context, from context to implementation, and from implementation to impact. The answer gleaned from the interviews was that there are conflicting views on private health sector growth: there are both proponents and opponents of privatization and user charges.

Proponents of privatization and user charges argue that these measures would contribute to a better use of scarce public resources and promote efficiency, enhance cost effectiveness, and respond to consumer preferences. Opponents of privatization and user charges argue that the public sector has been successful for many decades in Vietnam. User charges, as well as private services, could make health care less accessible to the poor. The argument, seemingly, is that negative distributional effects would outweigh any efficiency gains.

Policies on private sector growth in Vietnam are rooted in two issues: (1) How can socialist ideology accept private sector growth? (2) How can private sector growth provide both equity and efficiency in health care? First, the 7th Communist Party Congress paved the way for private sector growth by the adoption of the concept of a "transitional period toward socialism". Second, the 4th Conference of the Central Committee identified strategic measures to respond to emerging problems in the health sector. Among these measures was the diversification of health services, which was intended to enhance efficiency.

The policies for private health sector growth were conceived within the context of the polarization between rich and poor. In order to solve this problem, it is suggested that the government keep increasing its health budget. But, instead of using its health budget for subsidizing a large and inefficient health service system, the government should buy essential care from those who provide it at the lowest cost and with the highest quality in order to give it to those who need it the most.

In the absence of private services, public hospitals would not have to compete in cost and quality. Public health providers are opponents of privatization and proponents of service fees in public hospitals. In the absence of public hospitals, private hospitals would seek to maximize profits and this would lead to escalating prices. The role of public hospitals is to secure health care for the poor, and to keep service prices low. A diversified health system with a mix of public and private providers would be appropriate.

The key actors in policy-making are the Party (political orientation), the Parliament (legislation), and the government bureaucracy (execution of regulations and guidelines). The interviewees felt that political orientation and legislation are more needs based (more welfare based), while execution is more demand based (more public-choice based). The explanation is that the government is providing, rather than financing, services.

Within the Party, policy orientation is based mainly on political issues related to social welfare. Thus, the point of view of the health provider is not considered. Health providers have more leverage with Parliament members. Executive decisions are linked more with political orientation and legislation than with provision. At the level of the MOH, the views of public providers have more weight because of its dual roles, administration and provision of care.

These differences help explain why policy evaluation was considered of higher importance for process and context elements, but of lower value for implementation and impact. The other reason is that policy for the private health sector in Vietnam is quite new. There has not been sufficient time to evaluate its implementation, still less its impact.

3.6 CONCLUSION

3.6.1 The current situation

Vietnam is in transition from a subsidized command economy to market socialism. During this period of transition, Vietnam wants to make its health system more efficient. In the former command economy, public health sector services were completely financed by the government. Health services were free for every citizen. The health system was considered equitable and efficient. This is no longer true because of the high cost of public health sector provision, reduced budgets for public agencies, and an undersupply of public and private goods for individual benefit. The result has been increased demand for services from the private health sector.

The economic transition, coupled with urbanization, has created a rapid polarization between rich and poor. The health needs of the rich have changed and the subsidized national public health sector cannot respond to them. At the same time, the health budget is limited. The government should concentrate on meeting the highest-priority health needs of the poor. Responsibility for discretionary care must be decentralized. The development of private health services to fulfill these objectives should receive utmost consideration.

Policies for private sector growth could help make public resources available for treating the poor. It was expected that private hospitals would provide high technological care but the number of private hospitals is very small. The challenge is to promote the rational growth of the private health sector, focusing on the positive aspects while preventing the negative effects.

The growth of the private sector has helped the public health sector identify its needs: to enhance services, strengthen management, improve cost-sharing for public sector goods and services, regulate and enforce private health sector growth, and develop the necessary tools to assess the quality of care.

3.6.2 The future

The legislation implemented so far has addressed only the legalization of the existing informal private health sector. Why, despite clear government policy for private sector growth, has its development been so slow? The answers are multiple: the appropriate mechanisms for private health sector development have not been found; public hospitals compete with the private health sector to provide services to high- and middle-income people, leaving low-income people underserved; and resources are not available for the development of private sector hospitals due to other economic priorities in the country.

The solutions are not self-evident but might include offering low-interest loans to private providers, reducing bureaucratic procedures, and improving the management of the public sector (for example, by separating administration from the provision of care). Whatever solutions are found, the development of the private health sector in Vietnam must be carried out within the context of an integrated — public and private — national health system.

Part II
Demand-Side Issues and Lessons

4

Influencing Private Health Sector Growth through Financing Options

JAMES JEFFERS

Health Economist, Management Sciences for Health

4.1 INTRODUCTION

4.1.1 Purpose of the chapter

The purpose of this chapter is to identify major health financing issues related to private health sector growth. The chapter also discusses the advantages and disadvantages of some of the major health financing policy and demand options that are feasible for developing countries.

The chapter treats a wide range of financing and demand issues and policy options. Not all of the issues identified are relevant to every country. Financing policies that work well in some countries will not work well in others, and financing policies that do not work well in some countries, with adaptation, may easily take root in others. Thus it remains for individual countries to consider any policy in light of its appropriateness for their unique historical, institutional, political, and economic circumstances.

The chapter makes no attempt to develop an ideal health financing strategy for all developing countries. Rather, it attempts to provide information based on the author's observations and experience and on that of others (WHO, 1994). It is hoped that this information will stimulate discussion leading to refinements and modifications of issues, problems, and possible solutions. This process should result in a more complete understanding of the issues involved and the formulation of health financing policies that are appropriate for many different countries.

4.1.2 Major assumptions of the chapter

An assumption of this chapter is that one should not look at health financing issues without looking at the supply of health services. Health financing is not a goal; it is a means to an end: facilitating the provision of the types, quantities, and qualities of health services that are consistent with achieving national health sector goals. In addition, health financing drives health service delivery systems. The leverage effect of health financing is so great that it determines the structure of the health service delivery system, the types of services that are provided, and the allocation of health services within health resource markets (WHO, 1994).

A second assumption is that most health systems are mixed systems, comprised of both public (formal and legal) and private (informal and legal or illegal) health sectors. Public health sectors are command- or supplier-driven systems. The supplier, namely the government, is sovereign in determining what health services are produced, the terms on which they are available, and who is allowed to consume them. In principle, private health sectors are free market systems in which consumers are sovereign in making these decisions through the market forces of supply and demand. In free markets, consumer demand dominates transactions in the marketplace. Thus, if private health sectors were free, consumers would be sovereign and these sectors would be demand driven.

The experience of developed countries, however, has revealed that this is not really the case. Private health sectors are mostly supply rather than demand driven because consumers are not on an equal footing with providers in terms of information about their illness and the health services available to alleviate their illness,[1] and consumers have access to health services only with the permission of private providers. In reality, private health sectors, like public sectors, are more supplier driven than consumer driven.

A third assumption of this chapter is that, in the absence of policy intervention, supplier-driven private health sectors operate parallel to the government sector in a way that serves primarily the financial and professional interests of private providers. Private providers exert little or no effort toward the attainment of national health sector goals and objectives, particularly equity (universality in access to services). And whereas private providers strive to maximize operational efficiency, they are not very concerned about allocative efficiency. As professionals, private providers should strive to attain the highest levels of service quality, but they do so only on behalf of those who can afford them. In the absence of appropriate government-initiated policies, tendencies toward inequity and allocative inefficiencies are exacerbated as private health sectors expand and greater reliance is placed on them (Newbrander and Parker, 1992).

For these reasons, the appropriate government policy intervention with respect to the private health sector is to establish procedures and mechanisms for effective mediation between providers and consumers.[2] Mediation is not the same as financial intermediation, although third-party paying agencies are natural candidates for the role of mediation. Since providers hold the upper hand in health care transactions, medical costs tend to escalate more rapidly than is socially desirable. Mediation to

---

[1]See Chapter 2 by Rosenthal and Newbrander.

[2]In this chapter, mediation is defined as the use of an individual, agency, or organization that mediates between the interests of consumers and the broad interests of society on the one hand, and between the professional and financial interests of health providers on the other. This assumes that, in a purely private health care marketplace, health providers dominate the decisions involved in health care transactions.

reconcile these conflicting interests is particularly important for countries that are contemplating a rapid expansion of their private health sectors.

Health financing policies are important and powerful tools for accomplishing the required mediation. Yet health financing policies must be formulated and introduced correctly, or they can cause or exacerbate many problems, including undue cost escalation, excess utilization of health services, inequity in payment for services, and allocative and systemic inefficiencies in service provision (Parker and Newbrander, 1994; Akin *et al.*, 1987).

A fourth assumption of this chapter is the need for the integration of service delivery systems. Health financing policies and strategies must be consistent with well-conceived roles and functions to be performed by the public and private health sectors (Newbrander and Parker, 1992). These matters can best be addressed in the national health plan and subsequent deliberation and consultation. In order for the private health sector to cooperate fully, private sector representatives must play a significant role in this process. The process must be reinforced by the formulation and implementation of appropriate health financing policies that finally "bind" each sector to accepting and carrying out its respective responsibilities.

While appropriate health financing must incorporate payment system policies and mechanisms, provider payment issues are not discussed here because they are dealt with in Chapter 7.

4.2   THE NATURE AND IMPORTANCE OF HEALTH FINANCING

4.2.1   Financing, spending, and demand

Since most health systems are mixed systems, both the public and private sectors must compete for the available health resources. In the short run, the stock of health resources is fixed and the time required to develop them is relatively long. Training periods for doctors and other highly specialized health professionals are comparatively long. The time required to construct health facilities (hospitals, for example) is long compared with the time needed to build other types of service facilities.

Assuming that health resources are fully employed, increases in government spending for publicly provided health services result in increased demand for professionals and medical equipment. Increases in private sector spending increase the demand for privately produced health services and for the health resources needed to produce them. In either case, in the short run, assuming that health resources are fully employed, increases in demand will result in increases in health care costs.

In the long run, health resources are not fixed. Increased demand for either private or public health services, or both, will tend to stimulate growth in the supply of health resources, assuming that there are no constraints on factors such as production, training, and construction. In many countries, training facilities are largely owned and operated by the government, and medical graduates are required to serve mandatory periods of government service before being entitled to serve in the private sector. The time that must elapse before health resources can be committed to private sector service provision may extend beyond the period of required training.

Many governments, however, allow public health personnel and facilities to serve private paying patients, as in the case of Indonesia (see Chapter 11). In such systems, government health professionals play a dual role, serving the public sector during government working hours and supplying health services on behalf of private paying patients afterwards. In some cases, government health professionals are even allowed to treat private patients during government working hours in either public or private facilities. In such dual systems, as the demand for private health services increases, the supply of both services and resources can expand to a point where government facilities and personnel devote time and other public resources to the provision of private health services.

These dual systems present complicated policy issues, many of which are discussed by Rosenthal and Newbrander in Chapter 2, and in the country studies presented elsewhere in this book.

Given the importance of health financing, financing policies are key instruments for accomplishing desirable changes in the structure and operation of health delivery systems. A carefully developed and implemented comprehensive health financing policy strategy is essential to improving efficiency and equity in both the public and private health sectors; sustaining and improving the quality of health services in both sectors; determining levels of prices and costs for health services; and shaping the composition, size, and roles of the public and private health sectors.

4.2.2 Health financing and health sector reform

In countries throughout the world, the private health sector has grown in size and complexity. This is due to growth in household income, growth in private capital, advances in medical technology, and the emergence of social and private health insurance. More and more consumers are willing and able to pay for sophisticated health services. Within the region, there have been changing trends in disease and illness that have had a major impact on the age structure of the population. In spite of the growing demands and needs for health services, real spending by governments on health has remained roughly constant, or has even declined, in most developing countries due to slow growth in public revenues, competing demands for scarce public funds, and the comparatively low political priority given to health.

Asia is the most rapidly growing region in the world and probably will continue to hold that status for many decades to come. The problem for Asia becomes one of realigning the mix of public and private health service delivery and financing along more rational lines (Griffin, 1992). Such realignment aims to improve the efficiency, equity, and quality of services, with an eye toward greater reliance on the private health sector to finance and provide more health services than before (Creese and Newbrander, 1992). The exact proportions of public and private sector involvement will vary according to the unique circumstances prevailing in each country. This realignment of health policies toward attaining these objectives is often referred to as health sector reform.[3]

Table 4.1 presents several health sector reform options and a set of criteria by which they can be assessed: equity, several types of efficiency, and quality of care. The major financing initiatives (presented in section D at the bottom of the first column of Table 4.1) will be discussed later in this chapter. All health sector reform initiatives, whether they originate from the supply side or the demand side of the market, have critical financing implications. The criteria presented in Table 4.1 are useful for appraising financing policies as well. (See the glossary for definitions of these criteria.)

4.2.3   How much should be spent on health care?

Health policy-makers in developing countries often ask economists how much of a nation's gross national product (GNP) ought to be devoted to health care. Most economists do not have an answer to this question, refuse to give an opinion, or superficially discuss the pros and cons of the World Health Organization (WHO) guideline of 5 per cent. The fact that the question is asked indicates apprehension on the part of policy-makers about potential growth in health costs and reflects an interest in the need to control these costs.

With sufficient data and information for a given country, the estimated costs of providing a specified package of services can be calculated. The exercise requires that policy-makers specify the services that will be provided and that adequate data on utilization and the unit costs of service delivery be available. Those performing the analysis can provide a range of estimates reflecting best, acceptable, and worst scenarios. The expected percentage of health outlays relative to GNP rests crucially on the nature of the package of services, as well as on targeted utilization rates, costs and prices, and growth in GNP. Once these calculations are made, the costs can be expressed as a desired percentage of GNP. Unfortunately, in most cases, such calculations have little or no value.

The reasons that these calculations have little or no value are that decision-makers in most nations cannot agree on the most desirable basic package of health services for their populations; do not have the political will to attempt to control rates of diffusion of high-technology services, health care prices, and rates of utilization; and lack the institutional capacity to control utilization rates or the unit costs of production, and hence spending on health services. In short, the level of health spending is beyond the will and capacity of most decision-makers to influence or control, so calculating what health spending should be is inconsequential.

4.3 FINANCING INITIATIVES

Some may question why public sector pricing and revenue retention concerns are included in a chapter devoted primarily to financing private sector growth. The

---

[3]In this chapter, health sector reform does not imply that mistakes were made in the past. Reform is needed because significant changes have occurred in many countries and these changes warrant revising existing policies and initiating new ones. Thus, health sector reform seeks ways to realign public and private health sector relationships, strengthening selected areas of the public sector and expanding private health sector growth with greater efficiency, equity, and improved quality of services.

Table 4.1. Health Sector Reform Options and their Effect on Equity, Efficiency, and Quality.

Policy	Equity (access)		Efficiency				Quality
	Physical	Financial	Systemic	Operational	Allocative	Administrative	
A. Restructure health system							
1. Devolve management of public facilities to local government level	+	−	+	+	−	+	+
2. Decentralize health service delivery	NA	NA	+	+	NA	+	+
3. Transfer or contract management, ownership, and control of curative facilities to private sector	NA	−	+	+	NA	+	+
4. Promote cost sharing for specialty training and expensive medical equipment with private sector	+	+	+	+	+	−	+
5. Promote foreign investment	−	−	−	+	−	+	+
B. Improve public resource management							
1. Reduce public sector emphasis on curative service delivery	−	−	+	+	+	+	+
2. Prioritize and target public fund spending	+	+	+	NA	+	+	+
C. Establish level playing field between public and private sectors							
1. Revise standards and regulations	NA	+	+	+	+	+	+
2. Provide private sector incentives when necessary	+	+	+	+	−	−	+
D. Financing initiatives							
1. Revise public facility pricing policies	NA	+	NA	+	NA	−	+
2. Allow public facility revenue retention	NA	−	NA	+	−	−	+
3. Promote expansion of PHI and HMOs	−	−	+	+	NA	−	+
4. Promote expansion of community financing programs	+	+	+	+	NA	NA	+
5. Promote expansion of national health insurance	+	+	+	+	−	−	+

NA, not available; PHI, Private health insurance; HMOs, health maintenance organizations; +, favorable; −, unfavorable. Source: Jeffers (1995).

reason is that many countries have substantial public health service delivery systems with hundreds of existing health facilities and, for various reasons, wish to retain them. In those countries, the public and private health sectors are going to continue to operate in parallel for many years to come and thus are going to be in direct competition for health resources and clientele.

4.3.1 Revise public facility pricing policies

In general, revised fee and charge schedules should be based as closely as possible on actual costs. Since public facilities are government agencies, cost elements (for example, the cost of capital and depreciation of plant and equipment) not usually considered by the government should be included in the cost base. Numerous computer-based methodologies exist for allocating costs among the many different services, departments, and programs of health facilities, especially hospitals.

Given that hospital fees and prices should be raised, equity can be retained by the use of waiver systems, such as a means test. The means test need not be developed by the public health facility or even by the health department, but could be developed by independent agencies and involve members of the community. If a national health insurance (NHI) program exists, it could take the lead in developing an appropriate means test. Once developed and applied, the means test would be used to assess fees and charges according to the ability of consumers to pay. True indigents would pay nothing, those with ample means would pay full costs, and others would pay nearly full costs as set forth by fee and charge tariffs. Experience shows that considerable effort must be made to sensitize hospital employees, politicians, providers, and other members of the community to the need to raise charges and apply means tests at public facilities prior to implementation.

4.3.2 Allow public facility revenue retention

Public hospital revenue retention is a major issue touching on aspects of public finance philosophy and practice. Essentially, permitting public hospital revenue retention violates a basic principle of public financing, namely the avoidance of "pre-emption of revenue". While many components of government, such as tax collection agencies and customs departments, collect revenue, all revenues should be pooled into the general treasury. In this way, decision-makers can set national priorities and allocate available funds accordingly. If hospital revenues are retained and immediately invested in the collection agency, any decisions concerning the relative merits of alternative social investments are pre-empted. Nonetheless, pre-emptive revenue retention is public investment in the same sense as funding provided via budget allocation.

Departments of health usually argue for the public hospital's right of revenue retention on the basis that hospitals have little incentive to be conscientious about collecting fees and charges unless they are allowed to retain the revenues. Such an argument is weak because other agencies of government (schools, driver's license bureaus, and land transfer offices) have revenue collection responsibilities without the right of revenue retention. Admitting that public hospitals are not willing to collect revenues unless they are allowed to retain them creates the impression that department of health facilities are not willing to do their share in furthering the national interest.

At best, if the right of revenue retention is granted, budget and finance ministries are likely to reduce budget allocations according to fee collection. In such cases, public hospitals gain only by getting revenue more quickly than if they had to wait for funds to be released from central agencies at periodic and often uncertain intervals. But hospitals also lose: revenue retention rights (requiring an accurate accounting of these revenues) demand more work than remitting revenues directly to the treasury. Requiring accountability for collections makes sense because, once any agency of government is allowed to retain the revenues it collects, it is easy for fraud to occur.

The case for revenue retention is strengthened if it is presented in the context of a broader policy strategy, such as autonomy or privatization of public health facilities in the future. Granting hospital revenue retention within the context of a national strategy of gradual privatization is likely to be viewed more favorably by central agencies. They may even regard such a policy initiative as a desirable precedent for pre-emption of revenue by other operating agencies and departments of government.

Therefore it is desirable for department of health officials who want public hospitals to be able to retain revenues to improve the quality of health services. In this way, they can present requests for the right to retain revenues within a broad context of hospital reform, involving eventual devolution of management, ownership, and control to lower levels of government, or eventual transfer of many or all hospitals to the private sector when feasible. Feasibility depends on the financial viability and sustainability of privatized hospitals to operate without substantial government subsidies.

One potential source of financing that would improve the financial viability of public hospitals (Newbrander et al., 1992) and their eventual privatization is the expansion of NHI programs. If NHI programs are capable of providing a substantial revenue stream to public hospitals, it becomes more feasible to make them autonomous corporate entities or sell them to the private sector. Thus departments of health have an interest in expanding NHI programs while also pressing for revenue retention by public hospitals.

An integrated policy initiative encompassing both long-term privatization and health financing programs like NHI would allow central agency decision-makers to see an eventual payoff in terms of reduced demands on the national budget. Central agencies might be willing to invest in such an initiative so that public hospitals can improve the quality of services and compete more effectively with the private health sector and thus generate more revenues in the future. In short, eventual self-sufficiency of public hospitals with NHI and revenue retention as the core elements is a policy initiative that is likely to get more serious attention from central agencies and the legislative branches of government than pleas for revenue retention with no more apparent objective than getting more money for health.

The interaction between hospital revenue retention and NHI is presented in Figure 4.1. Starting at the lower left corner of Figure 4.1, the ministry of finance makes a contribution to the NHI program shown as contributions flowing from the treasury to the box labeled NHI. The NHI, in turn, makes payments to public and private providers, as shown in the right-hand portion of the figure. If government hospitals

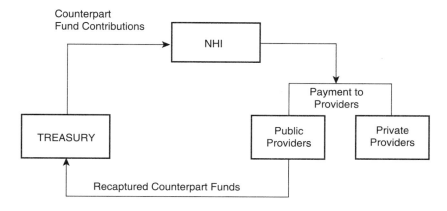

Figure 4.1. Recycling of NHI Funds from the Government Treasury.

are allowed to retain revenues from all sources, including NHI funds paid to public providers and user fees, these funds in effect revert to the treasury. Thus, contributions by government to an NHI program are likely to be recaptured, to the extent that public hospitals are competitive with private sector hospitals in terms of attracting patients and retaining revenues from charging user fees that cover costs, and collecting charges made to the NHI. Government reaches the break-even point to the extent that total user fee and NHI charge collections equal government contributions to the NHI program on behalf of the indigent. To the extent that collections by public hospitals exceed government contributions to NHI, the government would have leveraged its contributions to NHI and gained revenue with which to operate its hospitals. Calculations of NHI contribution rates, potential recapture rates, NHI payments for services, and levels of fees and charges under various scenarios could lead to decisions as to how best to make public hospitals autonomous. As public hospitals become able to retain revenues and revenues cover full costs, they are likely to begin inducing demand and otherwise operate in the same way as private sector providers.

4.3.3 Promote expansion of private health insurance and health maintenance organizations

The essence of insurance is risk sharing. The need for insurance arises when individuals are at financial risk for some hazard. Risk sharing is accomplished through contracts (in the private sector usually called a policy) between two parties: the insured and the insurer. The insured makes periodic payments, called premium payments, to the insurer, who is an underwriter, an entity willing to assume financial risks for the contracted price. In return for receipt of premiums, the insurer agrees to reimburse the insured up to a specified sum of money, or percentage of costs, to defray financial costs incurred by the insured due to occurrence of the hazard.

The value of an insurance contract to the insured is the ability to shift some or all of the financial risk involved in the possible occurrence of a hazard or adverse event to the insurer. For this right, the insured agrees to accept the costs of making regular payments during the time that the insurance is in effect. The insured buy a "product" that provides predictable costs (premiums) and other agreed-upon terms of payment, such as deductibles and copayments.

An important point is that people buy insurance only if they are at some financial risk. Since people are mortal and frail, everyone risks ill health, more so as they age. People are at financial risk due to illness, however, only if they recognize that they are ill and value improved or revitalized health status, there is something that can be done to treat an illness, effective health services are available, and they must pay for health services when they utilize them. If people do not recognize illness or do not see the value of treating it, they will not seek to consume health services. If illness is recognized and people know that medical treatment is effective but health services are unavailable or are available free of charge, or nearly so, people are not at substantial financial risk and hence would not be interested in paying for health insurance. Widely available free public services at low prices leave people with little incentive to buy either publicly or privately sponsored health insurance.

In the case of insurance, the insured pays for a product (protection from financial losses) whose cost must be reflected in the level of premiums. The insured should not expect to receive the discounted accumulated value of premiums back in the form of benefits. The insurance premium cost must include the potential financial loss, administrative and acquisition costs (marketing, education, and promotion), the carrying cost of money less interest earnings on reserves, and payment for the insurance service. Allowance also must be made for profit representing a competitive rate of return on the capital invested in the business.

Risk pooling comes into play when underwriters insure more than one individual. The probability of having to "pay out" to policy-holders because of an event of illness is very unpredictable, if only one person or only a few people are policy-holders. As the number of people of similar health risk characteristics increases, the variance of the probability of having to pay out for events of illness diminishes. There are also economies of scale involved in administration costs as the covered population increases. Thus premiums can be reduced as the size of the risk pool (the number of people covered) increases. After a certain size, however, decreases due to expansion of the risk pool tend to diminish and to be offset by other factors, namely increasing risks as existing policy-holders age and diminishing numbers of potential low-risk new policy-holders who can afford and are willing to buy health insurance.

There are markets for risk among underwriters. Some underwriters find themselves with a risk pool that is too high relative to the premiums charged, perhaps because policy-holders have aged, and increases in premiums could be competitively disastrous. Given that risk exposure is too high relative to revenues, an underwriter could attempt to penetrate new low-risk markets to lower average risks. This would take time, would be costly, and may not be possible. One solution is to sell off some of the risk to other underwriters who have a comparatively low-risk pool and are willing to underwrite higher risks, for a price. The sale of part of one underwriter's risk pool to another is called "reinsurance". Reinsurance is a common practice in the insurance industry and is done routinely in the interests of diversifying risks generally in the industry and thus lessening the risk exposure of any single underwriter.

As private health insurance industries develop, low-risk populations are rapidly covered. The populations remaining to be covered increasingly consist of high-risk occupational categories: older persons at higher health risks, people with pre-existing illnesses, people employed in high-risk occupations, and people who cannot afford to pay much in the form of insurance premiums. In the absence of subsidies, the growth of the private insurance industry slows.

In the case of low-risk group policies sold to firms, health insurance is so competitive that premiums are often too low to be profitable. In such cases, group health insurance policies are often offered as "loss leader" products to personnel managers who demand them as a fringe benefit to managers but are sold in combination with group life insurance policies or other insurance products that produce more cash for investment purposes than health insurance. If the levels of investment earnings available on revenues generated from premiums on life insurance policies are high enough, earnings overall are sufficient to cover health insurance losses and still yield a net profit.

Given the marginal and uncertain nature of household incomes in most developing countries, it is not surprising that private health insurance covers only a small portion of the population in which health risks are comparatively high. Incomes are comparatively low, and large quantities of publicly supplied health services exist. Given these circumstances, it is not surprising that private health insurance generally covers less than 1 per cent of the populations of most Asian countries (see Table 7.1 of Chapter 7).

Health maintenance organizations (HMOs) are comparatively new in Asian countries. In the USA, HMOs have grown rapidly because they offer a health care delivery and payment system alternative to the private health insurance that has historically dominated the American health marketplace. Members of HMOs agree to pay a monthly or annual subscription rate in return for the right to receive specified benefits directly from the health providers associated with the HMO. While there are many different forms of HMOs (such as closed panel, staff model, and independent practice associations), they all have certain elements in common:

- They are complete curative care delivery systems, offering outpatient and inpatient care along a well-defined continuum
- Revenue streams to the organization are fixed for a given period, and thus the organization is motivated to control costs in order to break even or make a profit
- Greater emphasis is placed on prevention and early detection and treatment of illness in the most inexpensive setting, such as outpatient clinics
- Greater discipline is maintained to standardize case management and treatment protocols in the interests of controlling costs. The fact that most HMOs involve capitated payment mechanisms to providers also serves to curb overutilization.

Many providers and consumers object to the "assembly line" standardized approach to treatment and case management adopted by HMOs. In many cases, consumers are not allowed freedom of choice of doctors and rely on their primary case physician as a gatekeeper to other services. Doctors lose some of their discretion in treating patients by being constrained to follow standardized treatment protocols and by having their practice patterns monitored by peers.

Technically, HMOs are not insurance companies, because subscription agreements do not explicitly transfer financial risk from consumers to HMOs. Legally, HMOs are regulated separately from insurance companies since, in the eyes of the laws of most states in the USA, HMOs are provider organizations offering quantity discounts to enrollees and are not insurance companies. Yet HMOs are at risk in the sense that, unless costs of treatment are less than total revenues, HMOs incur losses. HMOs have lowered rates of increases in health costs in the USA, largely through reducing rates of hospital bed usage and of surgical intervention.

HMOs operating in Asia are different from those in the USA. Asian HMOs do not impose strict protocols for treatment and case management, and statistical procedures used to profile doctor performance are not sophisticated. HMOs in Asia target workers of large firms and other low-risk, urban-based employed individuals and their dependants and do not include higher-risk groups. Most doctors and hospitals are under annual contracts for guaranteed volumes of patients, in return for which providers discount their usual fees to the HMO.

Together private health insurance and HMOs cover around 2 per cent of the populations of developing countries. Although the population coverage of HMOs is growing rapidly in some countries, such as the Philippines, it is doubtful that these organizations would be interested in, or capable of, covering substantial proportions of the population. It should be noted that HMOs and private health insurance operate successfully in countries that have NHI programs offering limited benefits to part of the population. For example, HMOs target Medicare members in the Philippines and require subscribers to make Medicare claims as part of the subscription agreement. Thus Medicare reimbursement becomes part of the revenue floor of Philippine HMOs and is taken into account in setting the subscription rates of members. Thus, private health insurance and HMOs simply supplement the benefits offered through established NHI rather than serve as a substitute to NHI. These HMOs operate in substantially mixed health systems; they are less inclined to price services competitively as alternatives to the fee-for-service system.

4.3.4   *Promote expansion of national health insurance programs*

NHI programs are government-sponsored social contracts written into law. The fact that they are written into law to serve unmet needs of society explains why they are often known as social insurance programs. NHI programs are often coupled with social security pension programs and other social programs.

NHI programs must clearly specify the benefits to beneficiaries. The beneficiaries either receive specified health services directly, or the right to receive monetary reimbursement to defray the costs of those covered health services. The financial terms of payment required on the part of individuals to receive benefits consist of premiums, copayments, deductibles, exclusions, and limits.

Most NHI programs are financed through taxes on wages and salaries, shared by employees and employers in the industrial sector, as well as civil servants. These programs cover employees working in the formal sector and their dependants. Much of what has been discussed in connection with private health insurance applies to NHI programs as well. They usually start by covering large expenses, such as inpatient hospitalization. Employees, especially low-income earners, usually prefer that money not be deducted from their paychecks. Employers also wish to avoid paying their share of these costs. Thus compliance, even in the formal sector, is a problem even when paid-up membership status is mandated by law. Enforcement of compliance with the NHI law is usually lax. Noncompliance on the part of firms is exacerbated by the fact that the benefits offered are often rather low, administrative costs are high, and enforcement receives less emphasis as administrative agencies become heavily involved in administrating collections, disbursements, and reserves as the latter reach appreciable levels.

A very important difference between NHI programs and nationalized health service delivery systems is that, in NHI programs, the benefits and the contribution rates are clearly specified by law. By contrast, public programs offer whatever services are possible given budget constraints, and consumers must accept what they can get from the system. In the case of NHI, people covered are entitled to stated benefits, which the administering agency is obligated to provide.

Because benefits, once granted, are difficult to rescind or decrease, social insurance programs are often conservative in their operations. Most social insurance agencies choose to provide indirect insurance (payments to providers) rather than deliver services directly. Benefits are typically low relative to revenues accumulated. These agencies tend to accumulate high levels of reserves, which goes against the principles of health insurance: if reserves are high, benefits should be increased or premiums reduced, or both.

Initially NHI coverage is restricted to populations whose heads of household are employed in the formal sector because collection of premiums is easy; incomes are comparatively regular; incomes of both employees and firms are high enough to support assessments for social security pension benefits and for financing NHI; and costs of collection and administration are low because formal-sector employers are usually large enterprises. Serious difficulties are encountered when political pressure is applied to social insurance programs to expand coverage to increasing numbers of the population, including those employed in the informal sector and the unemployed. Countries in Asia that have been able to enact universal entitlement are Korea and Japan. This was accomplished by enforcing grassroots participation through organizing local health or insurance societies, similar to the sickness funds that evolved in several European countries.

All successful universal entitlement NHI programs involve cost sharing among government, employers, and households or workers. Tensions exist between the government and other contributing parties whenever government attempts to lower the level of subsidy to such programs. Yet in principle, as private sector incomes increase and if the NHI program is operated as a single fund, cross-subsidies among private sector contributors will eventually suffice to allow government subsidies to decrease. Such funds do not attempt to offer all possible health services available as benefits, but rather define a basic benefits package for which the NHI is responsible.

An important difference between private health insurance and socially mandated NHI programs is that there are strong elements of cross-subsidy. In private health insurance, there are modest elements of cross-subsidy built into the premium and benefit structure; for example, young single males typically subsidize older employees, those who are married, and females in general because statistically it can be shown that on average they consume more health services than males. In NHI programs, by design the healthy subsidize the sick and usually the rich subsidize the poor. Social solidarity programs, including NHI, are usually "pay as you go". People pay when they can, usually when they are young and working; as they age and retire, the following generations are expected to shoulder the burden.

The social benefits of cross-subsidization also explain why membership in NHI programs is usually compulsory. One cannot allow voluntary membership and expect the rich to join and subsidize the poor or the healthy to subsidize the sick. In the absence of compulsory membership, the membership of an NHI program would likely be composed entirely of individuals with pre-existing conditions of illness or those who are poor, all looking for a subsidy, which probably was the case in most instances prior to the establishment of NHI programs.

NHI premium rates are usually established as a fixed percentage of a portion of income in the case of wage and salary workers, and of estimated incomes of the self-employed. Thus premiums are regressive with respect to income. Means testing should be applied in all cases of income workers, and premiums can be increased to cover all income to achieve equity. Thus NHI programs can and should be more than just resource mobilization mechanisms. NHI programs can exert significant leverage on the health service delivery system and the behavior of consumers and providers. For example, after the adoption of Medicare in the Philippines, growth in primary hospitals operating outside of Metro Manila was rapidly accelerated for many years. Health financing strategies, especially if they involve large NHI programs, can play major roles in positively reshaping the structure and characteristics of the health service delivery system. One thing is virtually certain: increased coverage for health insurance will increase the utilization of health services even with copayments and deductibles. This is because consumers will view the prices of health services as lower than before, and providers will be motivated to order or sell more health services. Thus mediation mechanisms are imperative.

Serious consequences can result if health policy objectives, the structure and characteristics of the health service delivery system, and the incentives NHI offers providers and consumers are not thought through carefully in the design or expansion of NHI programs. For example, it is believed that during the early years following the introduction of Medicare and Medicaid in the USA, they were responsible for rapid acceleration of health care prices and costs, with little or no increase in the quantity of health services provided to the general population. Whereas the elderly and indigent received increased health services consistent with policy objectives, other residents of the country paid a very high price in the form of higher social security taxes and much higher prices for health services. These increasingly higher prices have persisted ever since. An additional consequence was a significant transfer of wealth to doctors and hospitals, which absorbed the increase in "demand" presented by Medicare and Medicaid by increasing prices (in the short run, supply was inelastic). These negative effects occurred largely contrary to the expectations of many policy-makers and show that NHI programs must be crafted carefully and take into account policy goals and objectives and possible negative and positive consequences. Some of the issues that must be considered in establishing a NHI program are summarized in Table 4.2.

There is no single NHI organizational model that is best. Each country must tailor its own NHI to meet its unique circumstances (Normand and Weber, 1994). However, some fundamental elements should be common to all such programs:

- Establishment of the principles that accreditation is required for any provider to receive payments from the NHI funds, and that accreditation is a "revocable privilege, not a right"
- Establishment of principles and guidelines for providers' qualification for accreditation, including the conditions to which providers must agree to be accredited (such as possessing valid licenses and agreeing to participate in programs of utilization review and quality assurance, and to accept payment through mechanisms agreed on through negotiations between the NHI program and provider representatives)
- Specification of the types, quantities, and qualities of services for which payment would be made to both public and private providers (basic package of benefits)
- Establishment of procedures for monitoring and control of utilization (such as protocols for use of diagnostic tests)
- Issuance and enforcement of guidelines for the acquisition and use of sophisticated medical equipment and technologies
- Establishment of cost-sharing formulas for the public and private health sectors in the acquisition and use of expensive items of medical equipment
- Establishment of the NHI program as a single payer system that arranges payment for personal health service delivery, operating under global budget principles, regardless of the degree of decentralization of the program
- Establishment of an NHI program that forces cross-subsidization among private sector contributors, employers, and employees, with government also subsidizing the program in paying for all, or a substantial portion, of the costs incurred in providing services consumed by the truly indigent
- Adoption and enforcement of a national drug policy in which generic drugs predominate
- Establishment of guidelines for the eligibility of providers to receive payments depending on the location and level of service of all health facilities, both public and private.

4.3.5 Promote expansion of community financing schemes

People involved in community health financing schemes offer many strengths, including knowledge of local needs and conditions, enthusiasm, and, in many cases, a demonstrated commitment to the financing of health services.

Table 4.2. Key Issues in Establishing a National Health Insurance Program.

Issues	Factors to be considered
Enrolment	Voluntary versus compulsory enrolment (risk pooling, problems of adverse selection in cases of voluntary programs, virtues of freedom of choice and competition, individual versus social equity and willingness to pay, application of means tests to determine ability to pay, and social solidarity issues)
Legal basis	Regulatory requirements and laws and implementing rules and regulations required for establishment
Decision-making	Centralized versus decentralized issues (efficiency and equity: economies of scale versus "people empowerment")
Coverage	Horizontal coverage (percentage of population covered and entitled to receive benefits) and vertical coverage (the types of services covered and the level of benefits, such as support levels of benefits relative to actual costs of delivery, leaving remaining costs to be paid out-of-pocket by patients, and trade-offs between increased benefit coverage and cost of premiums)
Benefits	Benefit entitlement and portability of benefits across regions
Providers	Whether private sector providers are included and how providers are accredited with the national health insurance
Payments	How providers are paid and how claims are filed
Administration	Issues involving administrative efficiency (revenue collection, avoidance of fraud and abuse, investment of reserves, claims processing, setting capitation rates, and applying global budgeting as appropriate), mechanisms to detect and prevent fraud
Quality	Quality assurance and utilization review
Cost containment	Global budgeting; deductibles, copayments, and balance billing arrangements; and other quality and cost containment and efficiency issues
Sustainability	Policies on reserve levels and basis of premiums relative to costs of benefit payout and administration. How premiums are established and how revenues are collected through payroll deductions or member payments
Effects on the private sector	Implications for demand for health services and the response of the private sector (incentives for private providers to raise or reduce fee and charge schedules, induce demand for services in general, and incentives for consumers to increase demand for the consumption of health services

Community financing organizations have to consider the same issues listed in Table 4.2 for NHI programs, but on a much smaller scale. Unfortunately, community health financing schemes have fewer resources and skills to tackle these issues than national NHI programs. Moreover, they have many other weaknesses, which include lack of exclusive focus on health insurance; low levels of fund-raising capacity; poor management skills; lack of economies of scale in administration and collection and dispensing of funds; widely varying approaches to health financing in terms of benefits and collection rates; small risk pools with no opportunities for reinsurance, resulting in financial instability and consequent nonsustainability; and overdependency on the efforts of individuals who are not backed up by reliable support systems.

In order to further strengthen and support community financing, departments of health and other government agencies can assist local communities in organizing and developing their programs. Organizational efforts can be directed toward a large number of clients, including governors, mayors, and cooperatives, as well as toward individual communities.

A major concern is how to accelerate the development of community financing initiatives and to facilitate their broader coverage of people at local levels. Ways must be found to augment management skills, provide greater uniformity in health benefits, subscription rates, or premiums, and provide opportunities for the pooling of funds to generate greater financial viability and sustainability. This may require formal intervention by central or local governments. It may also require the imposition of greater uniformity on existing health financing schemes and on future schemes.

Consideration should be given to cross-subsidy arrangements that ensure that poorer individuals receive subsidies from those who are comparatively better-off, and that poorer communities receive subsidies from richer ones, under specified conditions. Such conditions should include complete registration of all community residents, issuance of health identity cards, and mandatory participation in making contributions to health insurance funds according to ability to pay. Meeting these minimal conditions requires acceptable means testing, accurate documentation of the utilization of health services by members of the community, regular collection of premiums, and routine and accurate accounting for premiums. Provisions could be made for communities to join together and form multicommunity health insurance systems that would pool funds, management, and other resources.

One approach that might be considered is to attempt to organize community health financing efforts at the provincial or national level. Comprehensive health insurance agreements could be negotiated between an NHI program and provincial authorities, such as governors. Mutual responsibilities for organizing, developing, and maintaining community-based health financing programs would have to be specified. Provincial authorities could be assisted by mayors of cities and municipalities. Such arrangements would facilitate the amalgamation of community financing schemes into provincial health insurance programs along the lines of rural health societies, as was done in the case of Korea. Community health insurance or financing initiatives could also be formally integrated into an NHI program that is devolved at least to the provincial level.

4.4 CONCLUSION

Most health systems are supplier driven. Countries must examine the ways in which the financing of health services for their system can be used to promote the interests of society for high-quality health services that are produced efficiently and distributed equitably. Such an approach can mitigate the problems of wasteful duplication by the public and private health sectors, lack of continuity of care within and between sectors, and use of unneeded services.

A major conclusion advanced here is that there is a need for mediation. Competition, natural or managed, is insufficient in health care markets to reconcile the conflicting interests of society. A countervailing power is needed to provide the required balance between the public and private health sectors.

NHI programs are the tools that offer the best chance of playing an effective mediation role in most systems. They are also likely to be more acceptable to all parties than outright regulation or nationalization of health service delivery systems, especially if the private health sector is involved in their establishment and operation.

Mediation performed by an NHI program can be supported by a department of health, a national health council, the cabinet, the president, or the prime minister. The most important factor is that one agency or organization takes a broad societal view in mediating among the conflicting interests of society as these involve health service delivery, financing, and costs. In doing so, that agency or organization is accountable and responsible for the nation's health bill. Close coordination must be maintained with the health departments that are responsible for the health status of the population.

All countries, regardless of the stage of their development, should carefully consider the benefits of establishing NHI programs. Such programs should be planned to cover the entire population within a well-defined period in a phased fashion. Naturally, the benefit package of poorer nations will be smaller than that of wealthier nations, but benefits can expand over time in a measured fashion commensurate with the rate of national development.

NHI program mediation consists of using financing and payment systems to bring about better integration of the public and private health sectors. Thus the entire health service delivery system operates as a unified system. Mediation can also serve to bring these two sectors together so that the comparative advantages of each sector are maximized. It should ultimately make little difference whether a provider is owned, managed, or controlled by the public or private sector. Rather, it is important that the health system achieves the production and equitable distribution of high-quality health services in an efficient manner.

REFERENCES

Akin, J., Birdsall, N., de Ferranti, D. (1987). *Financing Health Services in Developing Countries: An Agenda for Reform.* Washington, DC: World Bank.

Creese, A., Newbrander, W. (1992). Health financing and macroeconomic change in developing countries. In: *Proceedings of the WHO's International Conference on Macroeconomics and Health in Countries in Greatest Need.* Geneva: WHO.

Griffin, C. (1992). *Health Care in Asia: A Comparative Study of Cost and Financing.* Washington, DC: World Bank.

Jeffers, J. (1995). Review and summary of HFDP completed activities: technical implications, policy recommendations, and implementation issues. MSH Consultant Report, DOH/USAID, Health Finance Development Project, Manila, Philippines, 7 June 1995.

Newbrander, W., Barnum, H., Kutzin, J. (1992). *Hospital Economics and Financing in Developing Countries.* Geneva: WHO.

Newbrander, W., Parker, D. (1992). The public and private sectors in health: economic issues. *Int J Hlth Planning and Management,* 7(1), 37–49.

Normand, C., Weber, A. (1994). *Social Health Insurance: A Guidebook for Planning*. Geneva: WHO.

Parker, D., Newbrander, W. (1994). Tackling wastage and inefficiency in the health sector. *World Health Forum*, **15**(2), 107–113.

World Health Organization. (1994). *Evaluation of Recent Changes in the Financing of Health Services*. Geneva: WHO.

5

The Role of Health Insurance in the Growth of the Private Health Sector in Korea

BONG-MIN YANG

School of Public Health, Seoul National University

5.1 INTRODUCTION

Korea introduced public health insurance for a small portion of the population in 1977 and gradually expanded its coverage to cover the total population. In 1989, 12 years after its initiation, national health insurance (NHI) was born and the system is now fully operational. Along with it came a conspicuous change in the pattern of health service provision and in the composition of providers. The number of for-profit providers has been growing rapidly and they have become a dominant force in the health sector.

Health care policy-makers of some countries are looking for ways to increase the involvement of private providers in health service delivery. They believe that health services can be strengthened through the private sector by providing better access to health care, better quality of care, new impetus for innovation, sources of new capital, efficient use of inputs, improved technology, more responsiveness to the desires of physicians, and more consumer choices. Proponents of the private approach to health care delivery also believe that national health policy goals can be achieved through greater private participation.

Their basic contention — that personal health care is much like other consumer goods and therefore privatization in the health sector is largely beneficial to all parties concerned — needs to be tested empirically. Perhaps a *proper* combination of the public and private, with some regulatory features attached, could attain the objectives of a nation's health care system. However, a good example of such a proper private/public mix has yet to evolve in the real world.

Private Health Sector Growth in Asia: Issues and Implications. Edited by W. Newbrander.
© 1997 John Wiley & Sons, Ltd.

The case of Korea to date, unfortunately, does not validate the argument made by the supporters of the private approach. Rather, it shows that neither efficiency nor equity can be attained when the health sector is excessively privatized. It demonstrates that the type of ownership does affect the performance of a health care system. It could be a case study of a system in which under-regulated privatization brings undesirable outcomes as regards the public's health and health politics. Health care should be the right of all citizens, but this view has never prevailed in Korean public policy.

This chapter addresses issues related to private sector growth in health care in the Korean context. It briefly describes the Korean health delivery system and provides some data on trends in private sector growth. Next, it discusses some of the factors that underlie such trends. The impact of private sector growth on health care delivery is then analyzed. The policy agenda required to attain a balanced health sector is discussed, as well as the resource requirements and the processes involved in achieving this balance.

5.2   THE KOREAN HEALTH CARE SYSTEM

5.2.1   Health service delivery

The Korean health service delivery system has been basically a market-oriented, private sector-dominated, fee-for-service payment system. The role of the government has been limited primarily to the public health area. There has been very little regulation or monitoring of the ever-growing number of private providers to preclude excessive technology acquisition, excessive provision of services, unethical behavior (selective abortions, for example), fraudulent insurance claims, and income tax evasion.

It is a market-oriented system in the sense that health care is viewed, in general, as an economic good, but not as a social good. Access to health care is selective, guided by the willingness and the ability to pay. How much and what level of care one receives depends largely on one's income level. For example, there are the so-called special treatment charges (STCs). Thus, when patients prefer to be treated by regular staff physicians (board specialists) in a general hospital, they have to pay STCs in addition to the scheduled fees. If they cannot afford the STCs, interns or residents are automatically assigned to them.

The private sector, which was dominant in Korea before the insurance plans, has been growing further with the increase in per capita income and with the expansion of health insurance coverage. A detailed analysis of the private health sector in Korea is provided later in this chapter.

Patients pay a fee-for-service (FFS) for all services at all referral levels. FFS has been the dominant method of payment for physicians (both Western and traditional), clinical services, and pharmacists. (An experiment with a case payment structure began in late 1995. It is the first time that a payment structure other than FFS is being tried in the Korean market.) However, physicians at hospitals are paid salaries, and occasionally they are paid bonuses based on their performance.

In most cases, patients are given a choice of providers: they can choose among various providers at multiple referral levels. Because there is no patient referral channel, they can go directly to the outpatient departments of general hospitals. In 1989, some regulatory provisions were enforced in the choice of providers under the NHI. However, most patients do not abide by the rules, and hospitals, for fear of losing revenue, do not enforce these rules. As a result, the provisions have become ineffective.

Within the system, a "gatekeeper" — someone who could guide the patient to a proper provider or proper level of care — is virtually unknown. Since most patients prefer to be treated in general hospitals, both the outpatient and inpatient departments in general hospitals are overcrowded. Many local clinics suffer from lost revenue. Consequently, the concept of primary health care hardly exists. For many Koreans — and even for some health bureaucrats — primary health care is considered a synonym for public health or low-quality care for the poor.

5.2.2   Health insurance system

In 1989, the government of Korea launched a compulsory health insurance program for the entire population. It was the result of a gradual expansion of insurance plans from corporate employees to the self-employed and farmers. The steps toward expansion were taken without much resistance politically, economically, or socially. As of 1992, 94 per cent of the population is covered by health insurance plans and the remaining 6 per cent is covered by the Medicaid program.

5.2.2.1 Structure and payment.   In most cases, as mentioned above, patients are given a choice of hospitals and clinics. Providers are paid by FFS in return for providing services that are covered by insurance. Part of the remuneration is made by the insurance funds, and the rest by patients' out-of-pocket payments. Two types of cost-sharing features are incorporated into each service utilization. The first feature is a deductible applied to each unit of service. For example, a flat fee of about US \$4 has to be paid by a patient for each physician visit. On top of the deductible, a patient pays co-insurance rates of 30 per cent for clinic outpatient services, 50 per cent for hospital outpatient services, and 55 per cent for general hospital outpatient services. The co-insurance rate for inpatient services is 20 per cent across all types of providers.

Under the NHI, for insurance-covered services, providers (hospitals and clinics) are reimbursed according to a set of fee schedules. The government plays a major role in setting the fee schedules, although the level of fees is negotiated at the national level by all parties concerned.

5.2.2.2 Administration.   As of December 1994, there were 417 insurance funds. Each fund is financially autonomous. The size of each insurance fund is small, covering 30 000 to 200 000 people. With the current structure of a large number of small insurers in which each fund covers only a small fraction of the population, two problems arise. First, the system can hardly realize economies of scale; and, second, there is inequitable risk pooling among beneficiaries. The proportion of administrative costs to total expenditure is 10 per cent on average, and as high as 15.6 per cent. This high figure is an indication of the high degree of inefficiency compared to 1.5 per cent in Canada, 2.6 per cent in the UK, and 10 per cent in the US.

5.2.2.3 Coverage.   Not all health services are covered by the NHI in Korea. This is the most controversial part of Korean health insurance plans. The extent and the level of insurance coverage are determined by the government. Figure 5.1 shows the division of health services into insurance-covered and noncovered services, and their payments. Most of these noncovered services are new or expensive high-technology medical services. Examples of services not covered by the NHI system are computed tomography (CT) scanning, magnetic resonance imaging (MRI), most nuclear scanning, some chemotherapy, PET, and ultrasonography. CT scans were covered only beginning in January 1996.

In sum, insurance coverage under NHI is limited in several respects: the rate of out-of-pocket payment is still high, even with covered services; some of the expensive services are outside the domain of health insurance; STCs come along with both covered and noninsured services in general hospitals. In addition, there is an upper

Services Not Covered by Insurance	Services Covered by Insurance	
Market Fee (stated price of service)	Deductibles and Copayments (Cost sharing)	Payment by Insurance
Special Treatment Charges	Special Treatment Charges	

Note: Special treatment charges = Out-of pocket payments to provider beyond stated price of service

Figure 5.1. Components of Total Payments for Services, by Insurance Coverage.

limit on insurance coverage in terms of the number of days of hospitalization and care covered (180 days per year, 210 days for the elderly), including all prescription days.[1]

With highly limited coverage, most of the insurance funds have a financial surplus which is increasing year after year. By 1993, the accumulated surplus was 3402 billion won (the equivalent of US $4418 million). As of December 1994, the surplus was roughly equal to 2 years' premium contributions by all insured people in Korea.

5.3   PRIVATE SECTOR GROWTH

The profit-oriented private sector, which is dominant in Korea, has been growing rapidly during the last three decades.

5.3.1   Providers

Private physicians and pharmacists are the dominant providers in Korea. Although there are physicians and pharmacists in the public sector, their share of the market is relatively small.

There are two types of physicians: Western and traditional. Physicians in each category are trained by their own medical school system. They compete with each other for patients at all levels: the general hospital level (hospitals with more than 200 beds), the hospital level (with 20 to 200 beds), and the local clinic level. There is a third type of provider, the pharmacists. Pharmacists provide a wide range of health services by selling Western drugs and many traditional drugs, without doctors' prescriptions. Both Western and traditional physicians can also sell drugs for profit where they practise. Role differentiation between Western physicians and pharmacists, between traditional physicians and pharmacists, and between Western physicians and traditional physicians is not clear in Korea. All these providers have strong financial incentives to prescribe and sell more drugs.

Midwifery is another form of service provision, though the role of midwives is restricted to prenatal and delivery care. Most midwives are in the private sector.

Over time, utilization patterns have changed. Data (USAID, 1983; KIHSA, 1993) enable us to compare the percentage distribution of treatment by providers before the introduction of health insurance plans (1976), when some health insurance plans were available (1981), and after the NHI (1991). The following changes can be

---

[1]A prescription day is defined as each day for which medication is prescribed by a physician or pharmacist for a patient on an outpatient visit. An outpatient prescription day counts as a day of care just as a hospitalization day counts as a day of care. Both are deducted from the total days of care available for each insurance enrollment year. For most people, this means that their insurance will only pay for care for a maximum of 180 days in any 12-month period. For a patient with a condition requiring constant medication on an outpatient basis, the patient will use up his insurance entitlement in 180 days without any inpatient utilization. Thus, for episodes of illness requiring extended periods of outpatient visits and medication, the patient is at risk of not having sufficient insurance entitlement days available to pay for inpatient care if that person suddenly needs to be hospitalized. This provision of prescription days to define benefit entitlements is unique to the Korean system.

observed. First, there has been a significant substitution of hospitals and clinics for pharmacists, both in urban and rural areas. In the past, with low per capita income and no health insurance, people sought care mostly from nearby pharmacists. With the expansion of health insurance and the increased availability of hospitals and clinics, people depend more on physicians in seeking health services. Such a change is more significant in rural areas than in urban ones. Second, rural residents go more frequently to health centers and health posts (where community health practitioners work as providers) for their health services. This is a notable change for the Korean health care system because people now rely on the public sector for some services.

5.3.2 Facilities

Health care in Korea is provided by a mixture of for-profit, not-for-profit, and public institutions. Acute general hospitals, acute hospitals, and local clinics have been predominantly proprietary, for-profit institutions. However, there are some general hospitals and hospitals that are classified as not-for-profit. Many nonprofit hospitals, although legally so, are in fact profit seekers. Not-for-profit organizations based on volunteers and charity are rare. Because of public health and safety concerns, government ownership is typical among certain types of institutions, such as tuberculosis, psychiatric, and leprosy hospitals.

In 1977, the year when a health insurance program was first introduced, 53.2 per cent of all beds were either public or nonprofit (see Table 5.1). Seventeen years later, the share dropped to 23 per cent. Seventy-seven per cent of total hospital beds are in private hospitals. Beds in for-profit local clinics, whose number is estimated to be around 37 000, are not included in the private bed category. Lee (1995) asserts that if that figure were included, the share of private beds out of the total would reach as high as 82.3 per cent for 1994. In 1975, 2 years before the health insurance programs started, 34.5 per cent of all hospitals were public. In 1994, the share dropped to 4.9 per cent and the remainder (95.1 per cent) is now owned and operated by private or nonprofit organizations (Figure 5.2). Hospitals specializing in traditional

Table 5.1. Number and Percentage of Public and Private Hospital Beds.

	1962		1977		1987		1994	
Public								
National[a]	2564	24.5%	8504	33.3%	10 580	12.4%	10 642	8.6%
Local government/ nonprofit	3535	33.7%	5078	19.9%	14 759	17.3%	18 228	14.6%
Total public	6099	58.2%	13 582	53.2%	25 339	29.7%	28 870	23.2%
Private[b]	4378	41.8%	11 941	46.8%	59 841	70.3%	95 727	76.8%
Total	10 477		25 523		85 180		124 597	

[a]National encompasses national leprosy, mental, and tuberculosis hospitals.
[b]Private includes for-profit corporate, for-profit proprietary, nonprofit welfare organization, and private university hospitals.
Source: Ministry of Health and Social Affairs, *1963 Yearbook of Health and Social Statistics; Membership Reports* of the Korean Hospital Association; from Lee (1995).

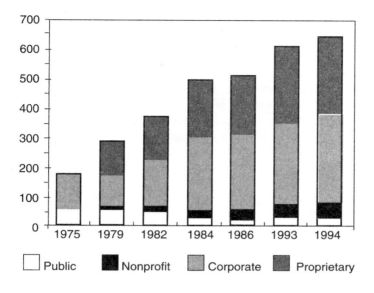

Figure 5.2. Public and Private Hospitals by Category.

medicine are not included in the figures. The shares of the private sector would be even greater if their numbers were taken into account, because most of the facilities and human resources in traditional medicine are in the private sector. The change has been dramatic, and the trend will continue at least in the near future.

Between 1982 and 1984, a total of 34 city and local government hospitals were transformed into financially autonomous nonprofit hospitals. The transformation lowered the percentage of public hospitals from 14 to 5 per cent. This change was part of the health policy-driven privatization that took place in Korea during the 1980s.

Since the urban areas have been growing faster than the rural areas, both in population and in income, the economic demand for health services has been rising faster in urban areas and the returns to health facility investment have been higher there. As a result, many private health facilities are concentrated in the urban areas, although this trend has been eased recently as some private general hospitals are located in rural areas adjacent to cities.

5.4 STIMULI FOR THE GROWTH OF THE PRIVATE SECTOR

Growth in the private sector has been spurred by many factors, some on the demand side, some on the supply side, and others on the government side. On the demand side, the rapid increase in demand for health services has contributed to the growth of the private sector. The increasing demand is attributable primarily to growing per capita income. It has also been affected by other factors, such as changes in the age structure, expansion of health insurance plans, a higher level of education, and people's perception of the importance of good health.

On the supply side, profitability in the health care market, more than anything else, has induced considerable private investment in facilities and equipment. With sizable returns on investments in health service provision, the private sector has quickly responded and filled the gap between growing demand and short supply.

On the government side, with the great success of market economic policies in the past decades, advocates of private enterprise have been gaining steadily over those favoring government involvement. Their ideas have influenced health policy-makers to favor private services.

Another factor that has contributed to the growth of the private sector is the philosophy underlying government health policy. Few politicians have emphasized the importance of equity in health care and the role of the public sector in pursuing the equity goal. During the late 1970s, the NHI was pushed forward by politicians simply because it was a popular political subject. However, they failed to fully grasp the interactions among the payment mechanisms, market forces, and the public sector's role in pursuing equity in health care. Politicians were not bothered by the growth of the private sector. Rather, some politicians, swayed by political lobbying, have supported a stronger role for the private sector.

5.5   ISSUES ARISING FROM PRIVATE SECTOR GROWTH

The growth of the private sector, in conjunction with the gradual expansion of health insurance plans, has resulted in increased demand for services and higher-quality care. The nationwide coverage of health insurance has contributed to increases in health service utilization and to upgrading the level of health of the people. The growing private sector imported new medical technologies aggressively and competitively, resulting in an apparent increase in the technical quality (see Section 10.2) of health care.

Annual health insurance statistics reveal that with the expansion of health insurance, the utilization of both inpatient and outpatient services has been increasing continuously over the last two decades, and that consumers, who believe private general hospitals provide better services, prefer care at general hospitals rather than at government hospitals or clinics.

However, these changes involved costs in the form of inefficiency and inequity, which stemmed from mishandling of the evolving system during the last three decades. As the market share of the profit-oriented private sector rose, many undesirable aspects developed in the system, over which the government has had very little control. Some issues arising from the growing private sector include cost increases, a two-tier health care system, commercialized health care, dependency on high technology, low priority of primary health care, and the lack of a referral channel.

5.5.1 Cost increases

Rising health costs are now viewed as a growing problem in Korea. The health care system of Korea is inflationary by choice. It is inflationary not simply because people demand more health care services, but because of the way the system is structured; it induces an expanding amount of service provision and consumption and, furthermore, of more expensive services.

Figure 5.3 shows that from 1975 through 1992 the health care share of the total economy has grown from a mere 2.8 per cent to 5.3 per cent, with an annual rate of increase of around 28 per cent. (Between 1975 and 1992, the Korean economy recorded unprecedented high growth rates. The increasing share of health costs as a proportion of GDP, therefore, signifies how fast the health sector expanded during this period.) Many factors contributed to the rapid increase in the national health expenditure. A substantial part of the total cost escalation is attributable to the increase in cost per case. The treatment cost per case has gone up 470 per cent for inpatient services and 240 per cent for outpatient services during the last 13 years, whereas the consumer price index has gone up only 125 per cent during the same period (KMIC, *Statistical Yearbook*, various years).

Increases in the cost per case can be explained by several factors: providers inducing more patient visits per case (supply side); more complex cases, and insured patients paying less out-of-pocket and asking for more expensive and presumably higher-quality services (demand side).

The increase in the supply of private providers, as well as the incentives created in the payment mechanisms, may have caused cost increases, as suggested by the data

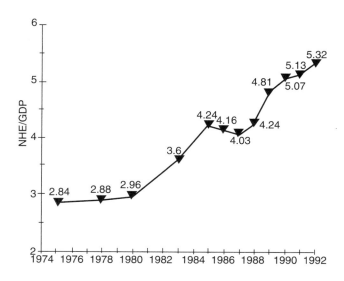

Figure 5.3. Total National Health Expenditure as a Percentage of Gross Domestic Product, 1974–92.

in Tables 5.2 and 5.3. Table 5.2 shows the difference in Cesarean section rates among general hospitals under different ownership. It suggests that because surgery generates greater revenues, private ownership has resulted in higher Cesarean section rates. The data in Table 5.3 on out-of-pocket payments for four major clinical departments in three types of general hospitals indicate that the extent of private ownership is positively correlated with higher rates of user charges.

5.5.2   Two-tier health care system

Korea has a classic two-tier system of health care, one for the rich and another for the poor. While some people can enjoy sophisticated, expensive services provided by private general hospitals, there is a group of people who do not receive adequate services simply because they are not able to pay for them. Those who cannot afford to pay the STCs, copayments, or the charges for services not covered by insurance, have to endure low-quality services. The situation is even worse for the public assistance Medicaid program beneficiaries, to whom care is often denied or who are grudgingly provided poor care.

Table 5.2. Cesarean Section Rate by Type of General Hospital, 1992.

Type of hospital	Number of hospitals	Total deliveries	Cesarean sections	Cesareans as a percentage of total
National medical center	2	1650	464	28.1%
National university	7	8253	2203	26.7%
Private university	41	68 494	20 548	30.0%
For-profit proprietary	37	22 831	8607	37.7%
For-profit corporate	55	73 995	29 154	39.4%

Source: Hwang (1994).

Table 5.3. Out-of-Pocket Payments as a Percentage of Total Treatment Costs.

	University hospital		Private hospital		Public hospital	
	OP	IP	OP	IP	OP	IP
Internal medicine	63.9%	51.8%	63.1%	50.6%	49.9%	23.6%
Surgery[a]	63.5%	58.0%	75.7%	54.5%	61.0%	38.3%
Pediatrics	70.7%	49.6%	83.1%	54.5%	55.7%	23.0%
Obstetrics and gynecology	90.6%	59.9%	93.5%	67.4%	87.4%	47.0%

OP, outpatient service; IP, inpatient service.
[a]Cosmetic surgery is not included.
Source: Lee (1995).

5.5.3   Commercialized health care

With the presence of strong profit-seeking private providers, health care in Korea is overly commercialized. Ample evidence of the loss of a medical care ethos and the gain of medical entrepreneurship is found in daily practice. An example of such a trend is found in the rapidly increasing rates of Cesarean section deliveries, which provide greater revenues. Cesarean section deliveries have increased from 6 per cent of all deliveries in 1984 to 21 per cent in 1994 for one insurance scheme (see Table 5.4).

Another example of highly commercialized health care is the practice of 1- or 2-day prescriptions provided during visits to clinics. This practice encourages patients to visit the clinic repeatedly for a single episode of illness.

Like that of many other countries, Korean culture has a strong preference for boy children. Korea's ratio of male-to-female births is recorded to be the highest in the world, followed by that of China (Ilbo, 1993). While the high rate of male births in China is the result of government policy, in Korea it is reportedly due to improved medical technologies and their misuse. Evidence of selective abortions is clear in data from recent years: a higher ratio of male-to-female births is associated with later births in a family (see Table 5.5). For example, in 1992, for all births that represented the first child in a family, there were 106.4 males born for each 100 female live births. But for births that year where the child born was the fourth in the family, the rate was 232.4 males for each 100 females born.

5.5.4   Dependency on high technology

Providers are keen not only to increase provision of noninsured services but readily invest more in them. A good example is the active acquisition of expensive high-technology products and equipment by hospitals in recent years. These acquisitions represent wasteful duplication of technology in the health system.

The diffusion of selected technologies over time is shown in Table 5.6. A significant jump in the rate of technology adoption is observed in 1989 and 1990, when the NHI was fully implemented. The marked difference in the rate of diffusion between 1987 (before NHI) and 1990 (after NHI) can be noted in the table. This rapid adoption of medical technology has resulted in Korea having more MRI

Table 5.4. Cesarean Section Rate for Civil Servant Insurance (Selected Years, 1984–94).

	1984	1986	1988	1990	1992	1994
Total number of deliveries	42 533	47 726	44 203	43 760	42 555	40 238
Number of Cesarean sections	2482	2619	4146	6067	7509	8356
Cesarean sections as percentage of total deliveries	5.8%	5.5%	9.4%	13.9%	17.6%	20.8%

Source: Korean Medical Insurance Corporation, *Health Insurance Statistics*, various years; from Shin and Yang (1995).

Table 5.5. Rate of Male Births per 100 Female Live Births, by Birth Order (Selected Years, 1980–92).

Year	Rate by birth order					
	First child	Second child	Third child	Fourth child	Fifth + child	Overall rate
1980	106.1	104.3	103.2	102.0	96.8	104.3
1985	106.0	107.8	129.1	148.7	143.9	109.5
1990	108.7	117.2	191.0	224.3	206.2	116.9
1992	106.4	112.8	195.7	232.4	216.7	114.0

These rates represent the number of male live births for each 100 female live births. The birth order indicates the order in the family of the child born. For example, in 1992, for all births where the child born represents the first child in the family, there were 106.4 male live births for each 100 female live births. In the same year, for all births where the child born represents the fourth child in the family, there were 232.4 male live births for each 100 female live births.
Source: Korean Bureau of Statistics, *Statistical Yearbook of Population Dynamics*, various years.

Table 5.6. Number of Selected Medical Technology Units, Total and Units per Million Population (Selected Years, 1977–93).

Year	Whole-body CT	MRI	Lithotripsy
1977	2	—	—
1980	8	—	—
1983	23	—	—
1986	73	—	1
1987	81	—	25
1988	104	—	30
1989	159	10	37
1990	227	33	42
1993	507	71	53
Number/million population in 1988	2.42	0.00	0.70
Number/million population in 1990	5.28	0.77	0.98
Number/million population in 1993	11.79	1.65	1.23

Source: Ministry of Health and Social Affairs, various years.

machines per million population than European countries and more lithotripsy machines per capita than the USA (see Table 5.7). Adoption of such technology results in cost increases for the system.

5.5.5   *Low priority of primary health care*

With the strong presence of private providers, curative care has been emphasized over preventive care, and specialist care over primary care. No matter what the

Table 5.7. Availability of Medical Technology, by Country.

	Number of units per million population					
	Korea[a] (1993)	Canada[b] (1989)	Germany[b] (1987)	USA[b] (1988)	Japan[c] (1990)	France[d] (1990)
CT (whole body)	11.79	NA	NA	17.7	40.33	7.20
MRI	1.65	0.46	0.94	8.03	5.91	1.20
Lithotripsy (ESWL)	1.23	0.16	0.34	0.94	2.30	0.60

NA, not applicable.
Sources: [a]Ministry of Health and Social Affairs (1993); [b]Rublee (1989); [c]Japanese Ministry of Health and Welfare (1992); [d]French Ministry of Health (1991).

physical condition, many believe — rightly or wrongly — that primary health care is a form of low-quality care.

5.5.6 Lack of a referral channel

The Korean system lacks a proper referral channel. There is neither a vertical nor a horizontal referral network. Patients have an unrestricted choice of providers at different referral levels as long as they can pay. They also have a choice among multiple kinds of providers at a certain referral level. There is no "gatekeeper" who could guide the patient to a proper provider or a proper level of care.

In the absence of "gatekeepers" in the system, there is inefficiency and a lack of cost effectiveness. Simple illnesses are treated expensively; for example, common colds are often treated by internists in general hospitals and simple headaches are treated by neurosurgeons in general hospitals. Moreover, patients often seek care from both Western and traditional physicians, and sometimes also from pharmacists, for the same episode of illness, increasing the revenues of the providers but not necessarily giving the patients the proper care.

5.6 THE POLICY AGENDA

The recent Korean experience shows that affordability and access are much affected by the growth of profit-driven corporations in the health care field. Health care has become a business. Providers refuse to serve those who cannot pay, will only promote services with a reasonable monetary return, raise prices to the extent the market will bear, increase utilization to maximize income, and aggressively promote excessive and irrelevant services that may not address patients' basic health needs but do generate profits. The very ethos of health care is being threatened by these recent changes in the delivery of health care.

Health policy will have to deal with these trends and the consequences of the growth of the private health sector. Further privatization, especially when it is carried to the extreme, will not be helpful in addressing the problems of Korean health care. This does not mean that curtailing the size of the private sector is the only option Korea has. Politically, downsizing the private sector may not be feasible, at least in the near future. Given the strong presence of the private sector, Korea must respond to two important questions: first, what is the role of government in making the private sector comply with national health policy objectives? And second, which organizational and financing mechanisms (such as health insurance) meet, or do not contradict, the equity objective of Korean policy?

5.6.1   Government health policy

There are two ways to organize the delivery of health care: government planning and cost control versus reliance on market forces and competition. Korea has leaned toward the market approach, with a two-tier system based on the ability to pay. As others have pointed out, the market approach is acceptable only when market failure is properly corrected by public policies (see Chapter 2). The behavior of profit-seeking organizations and the economically based ethic that emphasizes competition produce efficiency only if they are adequately regulated by market failure-correcting public policies.

There have been public policies to achieve national health policy goals in Korea. For example, the government tried to strengthen health services in rural areas. However, these policies were directed mainly toward public providers and the public health domain. In addition, there have been erroneous policies, including making low-interest loans to for-profit providers, allowing STCs in general hospitals, and offering little financial and organizational support for public health facilities. Little has been done to induce the dominant private sector to help achieve public health goals.

As a result, Korea has failed to ensure the attainment of both efficiency and equity in health care. In order to attain these goals, the government must play a role in making market forces work and in correcting market failures. Six areas of health care that are in need of strengthened public policies are discussed below.

First, the government has to provide the financial means that would allow destitute people who need care to obtain it. Korea has the Medicaid Class-I Program that provides free care for the poor. But only a very small fraction of the total population, 1.6 per cent as of 1994, benefited from the program, compared to the estimated population under the poverty line of 9.8 per cent (Park, 1994). Even worse is that not all health services are provided free to the beneficiaries of Medicaid Class-I and then only from those providers who join the Medicaid Program. Korea has no special programs for the elderly poor or for the disabled.

Second, a strict patient referral channel should be enforced for allocative efficiency. An increased allocation of resources for primary health care ought to be made. Also, since for-profit health care providers are keen to follow economic incentives, incentive structures should be put in place for providers to meet relevant goals for quality, access, and cost.

Third, there is a need for a corporate body to take responsibility for, or establish principles of management with regard to, technology diffusion and the utilization of existing technologies. Such an organization would ensure that technology assessment keeps pace with the introduction of new modalities of care. A health care network for utilizing existing technologies is necessary, at least at the regional level, so that the appropriate use of technologies can be ensured.

Fourth, there is a need for regulation of the pharmaceutical industry, especially practices such as pricing, marketing campaigns (which produce large payoffs for physicians and hospitals), and excessive advertising. Despite some of these practices, drug companies have brought major advances to medicine and their efforts in research and development should be encouraged and supported. A good public policy will guide the industry to fair competition, efficiency gain, and long-run growth.

Fifth, a public policy of defining the roles of the various health care providers is imperative. Lack of role differentiation among providers causes many problems, such as confusion among consumers, excess utilization, and cost inflation. For example, in prescribing and selling drugs, role differentiation between Western physicians and pharmacists and between traditional physicians and pharmacists does not exist. This provides a strong incentive for all of them to prescribe and sell more and more drugs. The result is that a high proportion of health care expenditures, averaging about 30 to 35 per cent annually, is being allocated for drug consumption (KMIC, various years). The lack of role differentiation brings about conflicts among providers themselves. An example is the battle in 1994 between traditional physicians and pharmacists over the right to dispense herbal drugs. This conflict persists and is not likely to end soon.

Sixth, some measures have to be taken to reduce fraudulent medical claims and tax evasion by providers. Government investigations show that both the health insurance system and the Medicaid system are widely abused by providers. Two policy alternatives can be considered: (1) change the payment and reimbursement structure from the current FFS to a form of prospective payments; or, (2) monitor claims and income reporting by providers more stringently. A prospective payment system (PPS), if successfully implemented, will not only solve the problems of medical fraud and tax evasion but will also have enormous impact on the incentive structure of the system. Because of this potential impact, providers in fear of losing revenues oppose it. Therefore, the adoption of PPS is not likely in the near future. In the short run, careful monitoring of provider claims and behavior may be the only plausible option for solving these problems.

In summary, the government and decision-makers should not view health care as just another marketplace but must intervene to correct market failures and promote appropriate incentives in the system for use and payment of services.

5.6.2   Health insurance reform

5.6.2.1 Feasibility of health maintenance organizations (HMOs). In terms of organizational changes to bring about appropriate incentives for both consumers and providers, one could consider having a payment system other than FFS. As pointed out earlier, FFS in Korea entails a great deal of waste and inefficiency. Considering the similarities in health care delivery between Korea and the USA, and therefore the similarities in underlying incentive structures and behavioral responses, the applicability of HMOs to Korea can be considered as one option.

One major obstacle in applying the HMO concept to Korea, however, is the existence of NHI as social insurance. Although NHI in its structure and financing mechanism is similar to private health insurance, it is still a statewide form of guarantee of basic health services. In addition, the role of government in health care delivery is recognized within the NHI. Borrowing the USA-type HMO (in the form of nonprofit or for-profit proprietary institutions) would mean a regression in Korean health care, in the sense that the minimal social responsibility that has thus far been achieved with the establishment of NHI would be abandoned.

One can think of a modified version of an HMO in which a regional government becomes an insurer, and public and private practitioners join as provider entities. It would be state-owned and state-managed care. Every citizen would be entitled to be a member through a compulsory premium payment. One drawback of a single HMO structure in one region, though, is the lack of competition among multiple HMOs. How efficient the performance would be and how well the built-in incentives would be kept alive in the absence of competition among HMOs are subject to question.

5.6.2.2 Expansion of insurance coverage. An alternative would be a reform in the structure of existing health insurance plans. As was previously noted, health insurance in Korea is distinguished by one feature: high user fees stemming from high co-insurance arrangements within the plans and also from full direct payment for noninsured services and of STCs. If equity is considered to be one important goal of the Korean health care system, the priority of reform should be to lower user charges through extension of coverage.

The three most important policies for expansion of coverage are: (1) to broaden health insurance coverage by limiting the range of noninsured services and also by eliminating the 180-day-per-year limit in insurance coverage; (2) to abolish the STC system completely; and, (3) to introduce an income-related co-insurance feature in health insurance, which would replace the current flat rate among all income classes. The strategy for comprehensive coverage and its possible outcome is depicted by three diagrams in Figure 5.4.

First, it is suggested that the STC system be eliminated. The major impact of this change would be a loss of revenue by most general hospitals. To compensate for this loss, the fee schedules of general hospitals should be adjusted upward so that total revenue for an average general hospital remains intact. The adjustment of fee schedules would be made in such a way that the net financial impact on general hospitals is close to nil. In Figure 5.4, after the change, depicted by moving from Phase A to Phase B, areas (1) and (2) would be incorporated into areas (6) and (7), without net loss to providers. Patients and insurers pay, in total, the same amount of money as long as consumer utilization of general hospital services is not changed.

However, this change is not neutral to consumers and insurers. Cost shifting takes place between patients and insurers: formerly noncovered charges (STCs) would now be covered and would be subject to the cost-sharing features in the insurance plans. Financially, consumers become winners and insurance funds are losers, although in the long run, all of the shifted costs will be reshifted, mostly toward the premium payers (consumers) and some to the government.

This change will bring about an additional indirect benefit, again to the consumers, especially to the poor patients who were formerly not able to pay for special treatment in general hospitals. With lowered payments for general hospital

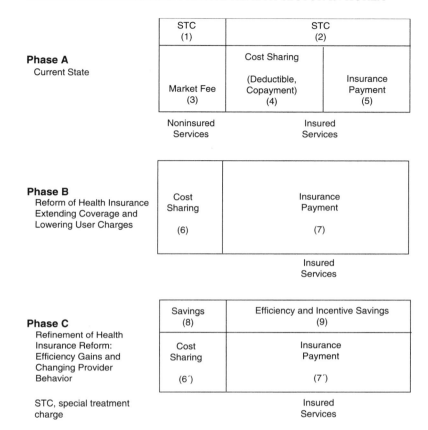

Figure 5.4. Phased Expansion of Insurance Coverage.

services, those in need of specialist care can have better access to it. Moreover, poor patients should feel less discrimination.

Second, it is recommended that all health services, except for cosmetic and beauty-related services, be covered under NHI. Traditional medicine should also be brought under the NHI umbrella, with some time lags and very careful preparation. However, priority should be given to comprehensive coverage of Western medicine, which absorbs the majority of health expenditures.

By adjusting the controlled fee levels, one can make the size of the aggregate pie that the providers receive (that consumers and insurance funds together pay) the same as before. In Phase A of Figure 5.4, the segmented elements in the current system — (1), (2), (3), (4), and (5) — will be merged into one and then divided into only two segments, shown in Phase B of Figure 5.4 as areas (6) and (7). The respective sizes of segments (6) and (7) depend primarily on the cost-sharing features of the NHI.

Through utilization of health services, there will be cross-subsidization among income groups, from the rich to the poor. The combination of higher (income proportional or progressive) premiums and lower (income regressive) user charges will certainly bring about monetary transfers from the rich to the poor, compared to the reverse case of low premiums and extensive user charges. The more direct user charges are replaced by premium payments, the greater cross-subsidization will be.

In sum, what the proposed health policies do is: first, bring most health services under the NHI umbrella; second, maintain the size of the aggregate pie that providers receive; third, restructure income-related cost-sharing features; and finally, make upward adjustments in fee schedules and premiums so that the system can be sustained. A major impact of this reform is cost shifting between insurers and consumers, which will make the whole system considerably more equitable than before.

After the health insurance reform, changes can occur in the conduct, behavior, and performance of the system as a result of a reformed incentive structure. The most important of all is a gain in efficiency through an expected change in provider behavior. As insurance coverage becomes comprehensive, the misleading incentive to provide noninsured services will be removed. Excessive adoption of some high technologies will be eased, as profit opportunities from noninsured high-technology services disappear. Ignoring the dynamic aspect of increasing utilization rates due to growing household income, population, aging, and other social factors, the portion of savings from corrected provider incentives is shown as areas (8) and (9) in Phase C of Figure 5.4, resulting in a reduced total spending of (6) and (7) to (6') and (7'), respectively.

Another indirect benefit of having comprehensive coverage is that health insurance can act as the basis for adequate government monitoring of providers. Information on utilization, revenues, and costs of formerly noninsured services will be revealed and readily available to policy-makers and researchers. They can be used as guidelines for regulation and be the basis for monitoring of pricing and supply behavior. Medical fraud and tax evasion can be checked with improved accuracy.

Additional resources are not required for the system to move toward comprehensive coverage, unless utilization patterns are affected by coverage changes. On the contrary, as explained before, there could be some saving of resource [(8) and (9) in Phase C of Figure 5.4] with reformed provider incentives. This prediction is based on the assumption that there is already a significant amount of supplier-induced demand in the Korean market (for example, 1-day prescriptions, a high prevalence of Cesarean section delivery, and frequent use of technologies such as CT scanning and MRI). A possible increase in demand from coverage change may well be offset in quantity by a decrease in supplier-induced demand stemming from corrected provider incentives, as long as fees for services are set at the right level. With the same quantity and lowered (controlled) charges, total expenditure would be reduced by (8) and (9).

Regardless of the cost savings, there certainly will be cost shifting from patients to insurance funds. Using Figure 5.4 and some supporting information, a rough estimate of cost shifting can be made. In the figure, cost shifting = area (7) − area (5), where the actual amount of area (5) in 1993 is reported to be 2775.4 billion won (KMIC and Federation of Medical Insurance Funds, 1994). The data reveal that the proportion of area (5) in selected general hospitals is about 30 per cent and 50 per cent for outpatients and inpatients, respectively. The rates could be slightly higher for services rendered by clinics. Another source (Myung, 1995) shows that in 1992, for personal health services, health insurance paid 34.2 per cent (2025 billion won) and the rest, 65.8 per cent (3894 billion won), was paid by households. Assuming the overall rate of 40 per cent, the combined amount of medical spending [areas (1) + (2) + (3) + (4) + (5)] would be 2775.4 billion won × 100/40 = 6938.5 billion won.

When all services are covered by health insurance with no STCs, and assuming the average rate of cost sharing, area (6), to be 35 per cent [that is, 65 per cent of payments are made by health insurers, area (7)], the insurance payment will be as much as 6938.5 billion won × 0.65 = 4510.0 billion won. The amount of cost shifting from patients to insurance funds in 1993 terms would be 4510.0 billion won − 2775.4 billion won = 1734.6 billion won.

This amount does not take the possible savings of areas (8) and (9) into account. When the savings from reformed incentives are taken into account, the shifted costs will be smaller than the estimated amount of 1735 billion won. Cost shifting, which might trigger an increase in insurance premiums eventually, is important to policy-makers and to some concerned politicians. Whatever the amount would be, extra spending by health insurance funds means that premiums would have to increase.

5.6.3   The health reform process

To realize a change in health care delivery, one needs the support of various sectors: the general public, providers, health policy-makers, and politicians. The easiest way to have a reform would be to have decision-makers and politicians develop a value concept about health care and have the courage to push it forward. Then, many of the current value conflicts and the confusion about the nature of health care itself, the place of health care in society, the role of health care providers, the relationship between providers and patients, and about whether it is legitimate to make profits from the misfortunes of the sick will be resolved.

Unfortunately, the reality is very different from this ideal. Considering the current complicated environment of Korean health care, it will be very difficult for the politicians and decision-makers to share their concerns and to act.

Providers, especially when they are private, pursue economic profits. The principle they follow is simple: they favor a change if it would bring about gains in economic returns, and resist it otherwise. They might follow a different rule if their behavior were effectively regulated by the government or governed by a different incentive structure. Otherwise, their choice is simple and unambiguous.

It is clear that the policy agenda proposed — tightening the government's control of the system and reform in health insurance — will produce benefits for the general public. The general public is likely to agree with the change, once they are informed about the background and effect of the change. Politicians may support the change if pressed by public opinion. Bureaucrats may back the proposed change once they realize that it is supported by both the public and the Congress. However, providers will be against the proposition. They will lobby both the government and Congress not to have any change. Eventually, the battle will be between the general public and the providers.

However, experience shows that the general public has been losing the battle. Either people do not have a consensus on health reform or they do not have an effective channel for their ideas. For example, in 1988 the government undertook an effort to implement a policy of role differentiation between pharmacists and physicians in drug distribution, making physicians the prescribers and pharmacists the dispensers. The attempt was a failure. Both parties, being afraid of losing revenues since they predicted drug consumption would fall with the new policy, flatly turned down the government proposal, leaving the public as the only loser.

Factors inhibiting public consensus on health care reform are multiple: lack of organization and funds, lack of leadership, the "free rider" problem, and absence of a core force. On top of these factors there is a perception gap between the public and health care leaders. The perception gap covers a wide array of issues such as what social health insurance is about and what to expect from it, how health care is different from other goods and services, what the health system is aiming for, and how the excluded population group is handled by the system. Therefore, what is necessary is the public's shared understanding of, and strong agreement with, what ails the Korean health care system. After that, a citizens' movement backed by formal consumers' organizations will help form a consensus on solutions for specific health care problems and express it to the politicians and policy-makers.

5.7 CONCLUSION

Korea faces persistent difficulties with the delivery and performance of its health care system, despite its implementation of NHI in 1989. Nothing is more basic to any government than ensuring adequate care for the poor, the elderly, and the disabled, and yet Korea fails to do this.

While the 1980s and early 1990s saw a rapid expansion of private health care, the story of the late 1990s is likely to be one of consolidation into giant hospital chains. This trend has already been triggered by *jabul* (business tycoon) hospitals such as Samsung and Hyundai Hospital. This kind of growth can only exacerbate the current problems in the health care system.

Korea needs health reform in many areas. In 1994, efforts were made to reform the health insurance system. Some minor proposals were made to lower the rate of user charges and to expand health insurance coverage. However, no one is certain if the proposals can actually be implemented. Even if all of the proposals are adopted, the user charge rate would be still so high that the objectives of the Korean health care system — adequacy and equity in access to care, income protection, efficiency — can hardly be achieved.

There are many aspects of our lives that are best left to market forces to determine without interference from government. Unfortunately, health concerns are not always among them. Consumer health and quality of care are neither protected nor guaranteed by pure market forces. No country has succeeded in having a sound health system by relying solely upon market forces. Some form of regulation of both the public and private health sectors is necessary, with the government and the professional associations as principal actors in the regulation.

Korea must also prepare for a new era as and when 65 million people, due to the unification of South and North Korea, together demand high-quality health services. Unless an enormous amount of additional resources is put into health care, the current system will not be able to handle the increased basic health needs. The current system should be overhauled for the sake of both efficiency and equity.

Korea missed a good opportunity to have a sound health care system when additional resources were pumped into the system by NHI. Now with NHI fully implemented and providers adjusted to it, it may be difficult to achieve even minor reforms. But, unless basic reforms are tried, resources will be wasted, consumers will not be protected, health care expenditures will continue to rise, insurance coverage will be reduced, and, consequently, the accessibility of essential care to low-income families will be further reduced. Without reform now, the problems will become more widespread, persistent, and intolerable in the future.

REFERENCES

Ilbo, Choong-ang. (1993). *The Economist*, October 3, 1993.

Hwang, N. (1994). Study on maternal child health. *Journal of Population and Health*, **13**(1).

Korea Institute for Health and Social Affairs (KIHSA). (1993). *Analysis on Health Care Utilization and Health Promotion Behavior*.

Korean Bureau of Statistics. Various years. *Statistical Yearbook of Population Dynamics*.

Korean Medical Insurance Corporation (KMIC). Various years. *Statistical Yearbook*.

Korean Ministry of Agriculture and Fishery. Various years. *Agricultural and Fishery Statistics*.

Lee, K. (1995). Expansion of the hospital sector. *Korean Health Economic Review*, **1**(1), 92–120.

Myung, J. (1995). Estimates of national health expenditure. *Korean Health Economic Review*, **1**(1), 1–29.

Park, S. (1994). *Estimates on Living Costs of Subsistence Level*. Korea Institute for Health and Social Affairs.

Rublee, D. (1989). Medical technology in Canada, Germany, and the U.S. *Health Affairs*, 178–181.

Shin, S., Yang, B. (1995). Change in service pattern under price control. *Korean Health Economic Review*, **1**(1), 53–73.

US Agency for International Development (USAID). (1983), July. *Korea Health Demonstration Project*. Washington, DC: USAID.

6

Private Health Sector Growth and Social Security Insurance in Thailand

DOW MONGKOLSMAI

Faculty of Economics, Thammasat University, Bangkok

6.1 INTRODUCTION

The role of the private sector in providing and financing health care is increasing in most developing countries, and Thailand is no exception. Private sector growth has been partly a response to the inability of the public sector to meet increased demand. It has also been affected by the government's policy of changing the public/private mix in the health sector by providing investment incentives. While public sector resources are geared toward the provision of basic health services, including promotive and preventive care to the population at large, private care tends to concentrate more on curative care, especially for those who can afford to pay.

Surveys undertaken in the 1970s and 1980s indicated that the sick relied mainly on self-treatment, followed by visits to private clinics and public hospitals. Later the occurrence of self-treatment declined and the number of visits to public health facilities increased, while the use of private facilities remained rather constant. In the 1990s, however, with the introduction of the Social Security Scheme (SSS) and the rapid growth of private hospitals, health service utilization rates and patterns shifted. Further changes occurred with increased demand and the expansion of insurance schemes.

The major demand-side factors include substantial national income growth, demographic change,[1] and increased education. All of these have contributed to the public's increased desire for better health. The double-digit growth rate in the gross domestic product (GDP) from 1987 to 1990 sparked off an increased demand for private hospital care. This was sustained by the continued high GDP growth at

---

[1]Demographic change has resulted from a decline in the population growth rate over time, from 2.3 per cent per year in 1980 to about 1.4 per cent per year in the 1990s, as well as an increase in life expectancy. Consequently, there is an increasing proportion of elderly people with greater demands for medical care.

---

about 7 per cent per year thereafter. With an estimate of income elasticity of demand for hospital care at about 1.62 and a negative one for drug purchases (Myers *et al.*, 1985), increased income leads not only to a more than proportionate increase in demand for health care, but also causes a shift in utilization from self-treatment to more institutional care. Moreover, a larger number of people can afford to pay higher fees in private facilities to have greater convenience of location and decreased waiting time for receiving care.

The increased demand for health care due to these factors, however, has not been satisfied by public hospitals, either quantitatively or qualitatively. This has allowed the private hospitals to fill the void. On the supply side, the Board of Investment (BOI) incentive measures extended to private hospitals have contributed to private sector growth.[2] The Customs Department has also facilitated private sector growth with a tax policy to exempt import duties on expensive medical equipment such as X-ray machines. Moreover, the establishment of the SSS and third-party insurance has enlarged the market for health services by extending coverage to low-income populations.

This chapter investigates the growth of the private health sector in Thailand and the changes that have occurred as a result of the introduction and expansion of the SSS. It presents an overview of the relative size and growth of public and private health facilities, including their regional distribution, types of services offered, and human resources available. It discusses financing and expenditures on health in the private sector and gives a detailed description of the SSS. It examines changes in utilization rates and patterns and, in the process, particular attention is given to the medical services that provide care to the insured under the SSS.

6.2 DESCRIPTION OF THE PRIVATE HEALTH SECTOR

Published statistics based on surveys of private health care providers tend to underestimate their numbers, compared with those from other sources. For example, according to the Ministry of Public Health (MOPH), in 1993 there were 270 private hospitals and 17 234 private beds.[3] Data from the Medical Registration Division, however, suggest that the total number of private hospitals and clinics with beds for admission was over 360, with 25 449 beds. While the published statistics may under-report the number of private facilities, they provide a detailed breakdown of the totals by type of services and by region, as well as comparisons between the public and private sectors. Hence, although the true figures are probably higher than those presented in the tables, this chapter is based on the published data.

The large increase in the number of private versus public health facilities between 1988 and 1993 is shown in Table 6.1. The facilities are classified into those with beds to admit patients, including hospitals and polyclinics with beds, and outpatient facilities, consisting of health centers and clinics.

---

[2]The BOI has provided investment incentives for private hospitals since 1973, accelerating its support after 1990. About 60 per cent of private hospitals in Bangkok have received some benefits through the BOI.
[3]Public Health Resources Report of the Health Policy and Planning Office.

Table 6.1. Public and Private Health Facilities in Thailand, 1988 and 1993.

Type	1988 Bangkok No.	%	Other provinces No.	%	Total No.	%	1993 Bangkok No.	%	Other provinces No.	%	Total No.	%
Hospitals and health centers (with inpatients)												
Number of establishments	116		866		982		155		1033		1188	
Public[a]	38	32.8	720	83.1	758	77.2	39	25.2	796	77.1	835	70.3
Private	78	67.2	146	16.9	224	22.8	116	74.8	237	22.9	353	29.7
Number of beds	21 685		66 667		88 352		26 967		81 401		108 368	
Public[a]	15 236	70.3	62 427	93.6	77 663	87.9	15 628	58.0	68 304	83.9	83 932	77.5
Private	6449	29.7	4240	6.4	10 689	12.1	11 339	42.0	13 097	16.1	24 436	22.5
Number of beds per establishment	187		77		90		174		79		91	
Public[a]	401		87		102		401		86		101	
Private	83		29		48		98		55		69	
Health centers and clinics (no inpatients)												
Number of establishments					18 136		4306		16 811		21 217	
Public[b]	57		8244		8301	45.8	59	1.4	9222	54.9	9281	43.7
Private	NA		NA		9835	54.2	4247	98.6	7589	45.1	11 936[c]	56.3

[a]Includes state enterprise hospitals; [b]includes health centers and community health centers; [c]includes 541 traditional medical clinics, 379 of which are in Bangkok. NA, not applicable.
Source: Public Health Statistics, Ministry of Public Health, 1995; Medical Registration Division, Ministry of Public Health.

6.2.1   Hospitals

6.2.1.1 Types and numbers of hospitals.   There are three categories of hospitals: (1) public hospitals financed and operated by the government, such as the MOPH and other ministries, state enterprises, and municipalities; (2) private hospitals operated on a commercial basis for profit; and (3) voluntary not-for-profit hospitals operated by independent charitable organizations such as the Red Cross.[4]

Public hospitals under the MOPH are the major health care providers in the provinces outside Bangkok. These make up a network of 17 regional and 69 provincial hospitals providing mainly secondary care, and 628 community or district hospitals throughout the country offering more routine care, which refer more complicated cases to the regional and provincial hospitals. Apart from the MOPH hospitals, there are public hospitals run by other ministries, such as medical school hospitals under the Ministry of University Affairs. Most of these non-MOPH public hospitals are in Bangkok and provide care not only to their own employees, but also to the general public.

The first four private hospitals operating in Thailand were voluntary hospitals. The for-profit hospitals evolved from well-established clinics offering outpatient services. They generally had a staff of expert physicians and the ability to pool financial resources; they eventually extended their services to include inpatient care. High rates of return on private hospitals have attracted more and more investment into the business, leading to excessive capacity and wasteful duplication. With increasing competition, business strategies have been employed to expand the market share. Such strategies include nonprice competition in the form of importation of expensive modern medical equipment, convenient location, and product differentiation emphasizing quality of services. Particular attention is paid to reduced waiting time, and amenities such as hotel-like atmosphere with attractive and comfortable rooms and fine food.

The number of private hospitals has increased rapidly since the late 1980s, following the economic boom from 1987 to 1990. In 1993, there were 1105 hospitals in total, 270 or 24 per cent of which were private facilities. Among these facilities, 44 per cent were limited companies, 42 per cent were polyclinics, 9 per cent were not-for-profit, and 5 per cent were registered with the Stock Exchange of Thailand (SET). In 1995, 11 hospitals with a relatively large market share registered with the SET.

Eighty-four per cent of the private facilities provide general services, and 16 per cent, specialized services. Of the 95 general and 20 specialized hospitals in Bangkok, 64 and 12, representing 67 and 60 per cent respectively, are private. In the other provinces, on the other hand, private hospitals account for only 17 per cent of the general and 56 per cent of the specialized hospitals.

From 1988 to 1993, the growth in private general hospitals was 5 per cent annually, while for public hospitals it was 2 per cent annually. The number of specialized hospitals fell, however, with the number of private hospitals falling more

---

[4]In this chapter, voluntary, not-for-profit hospitals are included in the private health sector because they play a rather limited role due to their small number. They have an administrative structure similar to that of private hospitals, except that the board of directors comprises the major donors to the hospitals rather than major shareholders. They increasingly function like private hospitals to ensure that their revenues from fees fully cover their costs.

rapidly than that of public specialized hospitals. The private sector share was 57 per cent, but the private share of beds was only 3 per cent in 1993, a decline from about 4 per cent in 1988. This is probably because specialized services are now offered in the various departments of general service facilities to provide greater convenience for their customers. The trend of private hospital expansion is increasingly toward the concept of one-stop shopping, where a variety of services is offered in the same complex.

The rapid increase in private facilities is more clearly seen in terms of the number of beds, which expanded at a more rapid rate than that of hospitals. Private general hospital beds grew at 11 per cent per year on average for the period from 1988 to 1993, compared with 1.6 per cent per year for public hospital beds.

The private hospital beds totaled 17 234 in 1993, representing 17 per cent of the total beds in the whole country. Just over half of the total private beds are in Bangkok. This number accounts for 40 per cent of the beds in Bangkok. In the other provinces, on the other hand, the share of private beds is only 12.5 per cent of the total.

Private hospitals are mostly medium sized, with about half of them having fewer than 30 beds. Only 23 per cent have more than 100 beds. On average, private hospitals are smaller than public hospitals, although the sizes of the former have been increasing. In Bangkok, the number of beds per private general hospital averaged 116 in 1993, whereas it was 414 for public general hospitals. In other provinces, general hospitals tend to be smaller than in Bangkok and the difference is between 49 beds on average in private hospitals and 75 in public hospitals.

6.2.1.2 Regional distribution of hospitals. About one-third of the total general private hospitals were located in Bangkok and surrounding provinces in 1993, and 26 per cent in the central region. The remaining 41 per cent are spread out rather evenly in the other three regions. This is in contrast to the distribution of general public hospitals, where 254 or 32 per cent are in the northeast alone, 22 per cent each in the northern and central regions, but only 4 per cent each are in Bangkok and the surrounding provinces. Thus, on the whole, public and private hospitals together provide a rather balanced distribution of hospitals, with the northeast having the largest number of hospitals to match its largest population.

The concentration of about 28 per cent of the total number of private hospitals in Bangkok in 1993 represented a decline from 35 per cent in 1988. This has been due largely to the rapid expansion of private facilities in the provinces surrounding Bangkok, namely Pathumtani, Nonthaburi, Samutprakarn, and Samutsakorn in recent years, following rapid urbanization and industrialization in these provinces. This is confirmed by the average growth rate of private general hospitals in these provinces at about 26 per cent per year from 1988 to 1993, while in metropolitan Bangkok, they grew at a rate of only about 2 per cent per year.

The regional distribution of general hospital beds shows that over 9700 beds, or 58 per cent of private hospital beds, are in Bangkok and surrounding provinces. This number consists of 56 per cent of the private beds and 70 per cent of the beds of the not-for-profit, independent organizations. With private hospital beds highly concentrated in Bangkok and public hospital beds more dispersed among other regions, the overall population:bed ratio is about 260 people per bed in Bangkok, in contrast to 1200 in the northeast, and between 600 and 740 in other regions.

In 1993 there were 40 specialized private health facilities in Bangkok and 76 in other provinces. As many as 74 per cent of these facilities specialized in obstetrics, 9 per cent in ophthalmology, and 7 per cent in dermatology. The number of private facilities specializing in obstetrics more than doubled between 1988 and 1993, reaching 86 in 1993. On the whole, there were fewer public than private specialized facilities, and the areas of specialization also differ. Taking into account only those specialized facilities with beds, there were more than 14 000 beds.

6.2.2   Clinics

6.2.2.1 Types and numbers of clinics.   Outpatient services consist of public health centers and private clinics. The MOPH runs health centers at the subdistrict level across the country outside of Bangkok, and community health centers in villages with poor communications and those located on the borders. Services in the health centers are provided by nurses and auxiliary health personnel, but there is only a single staff member in the community health centers. The Bangkok Metropolitan Administration also operates community public health centers in some subdistricts in Bangkok. They are located mostly in areas with a high prevalence of illness and large low-income populations.

Private clinics are operated either by a single physician or a group of physicians, some of them forming limited companies. The staff consist of one or more of the following: nurses, pharmacists, and cashiers. Clinics are generally open in the evenings and on weekends, since most physicians work in government hospitals during official hours and earn supplementary income in the private sector after official hours.

Polyclinics provide general as well as specialized services and are open for longer hours than clinics, some for 24 hours a day, every day of the week. Many of them also have beds for admissions as well as laboratory facilities, making it more convenient for patients to come to one place for different types of services. The trend is for many polyclinics to develop into small and medium-sized hospitals with an average of 10 to 50 beds. This has been a response to the increasing demand for private hospitals and the government promotion of investment in private hospitals.

The number of private clinics practising modern medicine more than doubled between 1984 and 1992, with an increase from about 7100 to 15 700. These clinics include medical, dental, midwifery, physical therapy, and medical laboratories. The published data for 1993, however, show a decline in this number to about 11 400. The drop has been significant for medical and dental clinics, while the number of midwifery clinics and medical laboratories increased. Several explanations are plausible for this unexpected drop in the number of private clinics: there may have been under-reporting; some private clinics may have closed or been converted into polyclinics with beds; or some of the clinics may have merged.

The average annual growth rate of private clinics is 4.6 per cent per year, while that of MOPH health facilities (without admissions) is about 1.3 per cent per year.

In addition to modern medical clinics, there were 541 traditional medical and midwifery clinics across the country in 1993. The majority of these clinics are in Bangkok and the central region. It seems that traditional medicine is slowly reviving in popularity among the Thai population, as university departments and research institutes in medical sciences pay more attention to the study of traditional medicine. The price of traditional medicine is also much lower than that of modern medicine.

6.2.2.2 Regional distribution of clinics.   The regional distribution of clinics is similar to that of private hospitals, with private clinics located primarily in Bangkok and other urban areas. About one-third of the total are in Bangkok, 18 per cent each in the central and northern regions, and only 15 per cent in the south.

6.2.3   Pharmacies

6.2.3.1 Types and numbers of pharmacies.   Another type of private health facility, which is very popular, is the pharmacy. A large proportion of household expenditures on medical care goes to the purchase of drugs from pharmacies. Although this proportion has declined over time, as preference shifts to institutional care in hospitals and clinics, about 20 per cent of medical care expenditures are still allocated to drug purchases from this source.

In early 1994, there were almost 10 000 modern pharmacies and over 2000 traditional pharmacies across the country. About 45 per cent of the modern pharmacies are Type I, having a license to sell all modern drugs, and the rest are Type II, having a license to sell only ready-packed drugs that are not dangerous or specially controlled.

6.2.3.2 Regional distribution of pharmacies.   The majority of the Type I pharmacies are located in Bangkok (48 per cent) and the central region (24 per cent), while most of the Type II pharmacies are more evenly distributed in the regions: central (30 per cent), northeast (23 per cent), and northern (21 per cent). Traditional pharmacies are also highest in number in the central region (29 per cent) and the northeast region (27 per cent).

6.2.4   Providers

6.2.4.1 Types and numbers of providers.   Most medical personnel, particularly doctors, have their main jobs in the public sector, and either operate their own clinics or practise in private hospitals in the evenings and on weekends. A study by Chunharas *et al.* (1992) indicates that a general practitioner in regional and general hospitals and medical schools in Bangkok works on average 69.6 h per week, 46 h in the regular or primary job and 23.6 h in a supplemental job. A specialist in orthopedic surgery, for example, has an average work week of 75.6 h, of which 57.5 h are accounted for by their primary job.

Thus, to obtain an accurate full-time equivalent number of doctors in the private sector, assuming that about 80 per cent of the doctors in the public sector have supplemental private practices, and that doctors work in those jobs about one-third

Table 6.2. Health Human Resources, Number and Distribution by Category, 1993.

	Bangkok		Other provinces			Percentage in private sector
	No.	%	No.	%	Total	
Physician	6191	45.4	7443	54.6	13634	18.6
Population per physician	900	–	7055	–	4260	–
Dentist	1331	47.8	1455	52.2	2786	23.5
Population per dentist	4183	–	36079	–	20841	–
Pharmacist	2717	57.6	2004	42.4	4721	35.7
Population per pharmacist	2049	–	26195	–	12229	–
Nurse	17334	23.5	56350	76.5	73684	10.4
Population per nurse	321	–	932	–	788	–
Midwife	375	3.6	10150	96.4	10525	4.2
Population per midwife	14690	–	5174	–	5517	–

Source: Public Health Statistics, Ministry of Public Health, 1995; Drug Control Division, The Food and Drug Administration, Ministry of Public Health.

as much as they work in the public sector, approximately 26 per cent of the number of doctors in the public sector should be added to that in the private sector.

The number of all providers working in the private sector (except midwives) has increased. The rapid increase is attributable to the intensified demand for providers to operate the new private hospitals. Between 1988 and 1993, the percentages of doctors and auxiliary nurses employed in the private sector have nearly doubled, while those of other types of medical personnel increased by less. On the other hand, the proportion of pharmacists in the private sector has declined. A shortage of pharmacists has been reported in 98 per cent of the pharmaceutical production companies.[5]

The supply of providers has been increasing rapidly because of the expanded capacity of medical and nursing schools to produce graduates. This had led to an improvement in the population:provider ratios over time.

6.2.4.2 Regional distribution of health personnel. There is a maldistribution of health personnel between Bangkok and the other provinces (see Table 6.2). About 45 per cent of the physicians are in Bangkok, taking care of about 14 per cent of the population. Hence, the population:physician ratio is 900 in Bangkok, but in other provinces the ratio is over 7000.

Of the 13000 specialist physicians (about 3000 general practitioners), almost 30 per cent are in Bangkok and 20 per cent in the private sector. Specialists tend to be more concentrated in Bangkok than general practitioners. For most areas of specialization, more than half of the physicians are in Bangkok and an average of 19 per cent are in the private sector.

There is maldistribution, with other health personnel being concentrated in Bangkok as well: 48 per cent of dentists, 58 per cent of pharmacists, and 24 per cent

[5]These data come from a survey conducted by the Thai Pharmaceuticals Manufacturers Association in 1992.

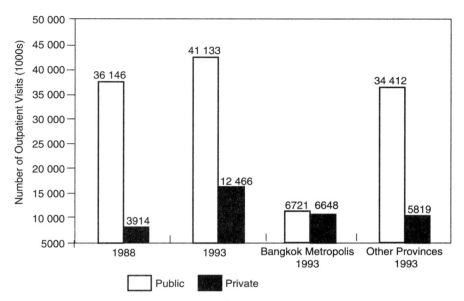

Figure 6.1. Outpatient Visits, 1988 and 1993.

of nurses. Consequently, population:provider ratios differ greatly between Bangkok and other provinces. Among regions, the northeast has the worst ratio, with one doctor for over 10 000 people, one dentist for 50 000, one pharmacist for 42 000, and one nurse for 1400.

Not surprisingly, there is no significant shortage of providers in large urban areas, particularly Bangkok, while the numbers in the rural areas are inadequate. However, in Bangkok there have been significant transfers of medical personnel from the public to the private sector in recent years due to rapid private sector growth and the large discrepancy in salaries offered by the public and private sectors. This has caused shortages in certain parts of the public sector, particularly in small hospitals and those located outside the city.

6.3   UTILIZATION OF PRIVATE HEALTH FACILITIES

The total number of outpatients using general health facilities increased over time, from 17.4 million in 1988 to 19.6 million in 1993, and that of inpatients from 3.7 million to 4.8 million in the same period. Private facilities have had a larger increase in utilization by both outpatients and inpatients than public facilities. In addition to serving domestic users, private hospitals in the large cities in each region also serve an increasing number of users from other Asian countries. Some private hospitals in Bangkok also set up centers to treat foreign patients.

Between 1988 and 1993, the number of outpatient visits to private general facilities more than tripled, from 3.9 million to 12.5 million, while that in public facilities increased by only 5 million, from 36.1 million to 41.1 million (see Figure 6.1).

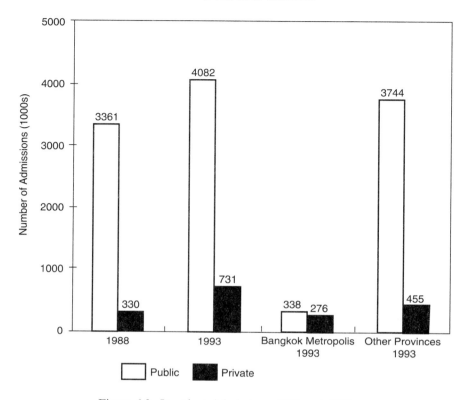

Figure 6.2. Inpatient Admissions, 1988 and 1993.

Consequently, the share of private facilities for outpatient visits more than doubled, from 10 per cent to 23 per cent. This is because average outpatient visits increased significantly, from 1.5 visits per patient in 1988 to 4.1 visits in 1993. It is not known if these are increases in first visits or a volume increase in follow-up consultations. Greater accessibility to private facilities, especially in Bangkok and other large urban areas, has probably been responsible for most of the increase in the number of outpatient visits per patient. The increase in average visits could also have been supplier induced.

Like outpatient visits, inpatient admissions to private facilities increased from 9 per cent to 15 per cent between 1988 and 1993 (see Figure 6.2). This is a result of the rapid annual growth rate in utilization of private inpatient facilities of about 20 per cent per year on average for the number of inpatients, and 6 per cent per year for inpatient days, compared to 4 and 3 per cent respectively for public hospitals.

Although the total number of inpatient days increased, the average length of stay in private facilities dropped sharply from 5.8 to 3.5 days between 1988 and 1993 (see Figure 6.3). Public facilities experienced a small decline, from 5.0 to 4.8 days. This difference was due mainly to much higher charges in private facilities and the limited reimbursement of medical care expenditures allowed by a number of health

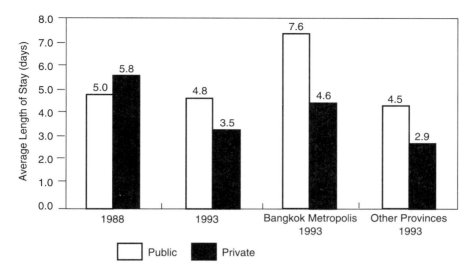

Figure 6.3. Average Length of Hospital Stay, 1988 and 1993.

insurance schemes for services received in private hospitals, such as the Civil Servants' Medical Benefit Scheme.

Utilization of private specialized facilities, on the other hand, has shown a significant decline. Consequently, private sector shares of the number of patients, the number of outpatient visits, and inpatient days have fallen between 1988 and 1993. In 1993, utilization of public specialized facilities was over 95 per cent of the total. This trend could be explained by a shift toward greater utilization of general private facilities as the number and beds of these facilities expanded and those of specialized facilities decreased.

There seems to be a clear market segmentation between public and private hospitals according to demographic and geographic factors. The market opportunities for private hospitals lie in providing services to the elderly, those entering the labor force, those in higher-income groups, and those living in urban areas. Public hospitals, on the other hand, serve the low-income populations, mostly in the rural areas.

6.4   HEALTH FINANCING AND HOUSEHOLD HEALTH CARE EXPENDITURE

Total health care expenditure in Thailand accounts for nearly 6 per cent of GDP. Per capita expenditure was about 2500 baht in 1992 (US $1 = 25 baht). Households and private companies have been contributing about 70 per cent of the total health care expenditure and this proportion has increased over time. On the other hand, public sources of finance — mainly from the MOPH — have declined.

Table 6.3. Summary of Financing Schemes, 1993.

Scheme	Nature of scheme	Population covered (no. and %)	Source of funds	Expenditure per capita (baht)
Free medical care	Social welfare	Low income 11.7 million / Elderly 3.5 million / Primary school children 5.1 million (35.9%)	General tax	214 / 72 / 31
Civil Servants and State Enterprises Medical Benefit	Public employee fringe benefits	Employees, pensioners, 6.4 million and dependants (11.3%)	General tax	916
Social Security	Compulsory health insurance for firms with more than 10 employees	Employees 4.6 million (8.1%)	Tripartite	805
Workmen's Compensation Fund		Employees 1.8 million	Employer	421
Health cards	Voluntary health insurance	1.3 million (2.3%)	Household and general tax	141
Private health insurance		0.9 million (1.6%)	Household	933
Total covered population		59.2%		

Low income: monthly income below 2800 baht for households and 2000 for singles; elderly: population 60 years old and above.
Source: Compiled from papers presented at the national workshop "Health Financing in Thailand", November 12–13 1993, Phetburi.

Various financing schemes for health care exist in Thailand, covering almost 60 per cent of the total population. Some of these schemes are voluntary, some are compulsory, and some are fringe benefits and social welfare schemes. Table 6.3 provides a summary of these schemes and their major characteristics, showing that all the schemes covered about 35 million or 59 per cent of the total population in 1993.

These financing schemes vary greatly in terms of their target groups, population coverage, benefits, choice of providers, and source of funds, as well as the payment mechanisms and expenditures involved. Some of them, such as the SSS and the Workmen's Compensation Scheme (WCS), extend complementary benefits to the same population group but use different payment mechanisms. Such diverse and fragmented approaches to providing health benefits create inefficiencies and inequities among the 59 per cent of the population covered by some benefit scheme, as well as between those covered and the remaining 41 per cent not covered by any scheme. Those not covered by some scheme include rural agricultural workers, urban street vendors, the self-employed, and others engaged in informal activities.

The government totally finances the Civil Servants and State Enterprises Medical Benefit Schemes. These schemes, which provide free health care as fringe benefits to current civil servants and state enterprise employees, pensioners, and dependants, cover 11 per cent of the population. The government also finances, as a social welfare program, free health care for the poor, the elderly, the handicapped, and children under 12 years. This program provides the largest population coverage, 36 per cent.

The government partially subsidizes the SSS (see below). Since 1994, the health card program, which is a voluntary insurance scheme for rural populations, has had an equal matching fund of 500 baht per card from the government. These two schemes cover another 10 per cent of the population.

The major sources of expenditure, accounting for over 70 per cent of total health care expenditure, are private employers and households. Private employers contribute another one-third to the Social Security Fund and totally finance the Workmen's Compensation Fund to provide health benefits for work-related injuries or illnesses of their employees. Households provide out-of-pocket payments, including one-third of employees' contribution to the Social Security Fund, payment for the purchase of health cards and private health insurance premiums, and self-financing of the health expenses incurred when they seek care.

According to data from the 1992 Socio-Economic Surveys, households spend an average of 226 baht per month on health care. This amount is about 5.7 per cent of their total monthly expenditure or 4.1 per cent of their monthly money income. The amount is divided between 17 per cent spent on medicine and supplies purchased from pharmacies for self-treatment, and 83 per cent on health services and drugs purchased by prescription from health facilities. Of the health services expenditure, 43 per cent is paid for services received in private hospitals and clinics, 34 per cent for government hospital services, 4 per cent for doctor and dentist fees, and the remainder for eye examinations, nurses and midwives, and other services. The amount spent on private facilities may be accounted for by price differentials rather than increased volume, since it has been reported that the private sector charges two

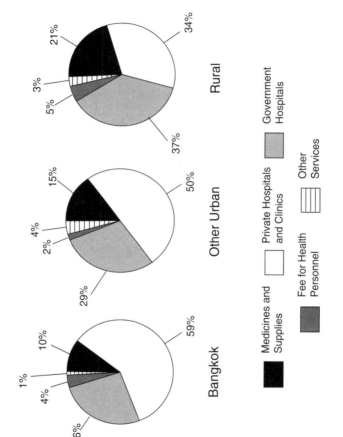

Figure 6.4. Average Monthly Household Expenditure on Health Care in 1992.

to three times more than public hospitals for diagnostic laboratory tests and X-rays, and about five to ten times more for room charges. Figure 6.4 shows the differences in the proportion of health services expenditure spent on self-purchased drugs and institutional care for households in Bangkok, other urban areas, and rural areas in 1992.

When the 1992 survey data are compared with those of 1988 and 1990, it is found that expenditure on health services increased in real terms over time but those on drugs remained stable. Health services expenditure at private hospitals and clinics increased the most. Health care expenditure spent on self-purchased drugs declined from 22 per cent in 1988 to 19 per cent in 1990 to 17 per cent in 1992. As for health services expenditure, the proportion spent on private facilities increased over time at the expense of self-purchased drugs.

6.5   THE SOCIAL SECURITY SCHEME

The SSS and the WCS are compulsory insurance for employees working in business enterprises with 10 or more employees. These schemes cover almost 8 per cent of the population.

Before the enactment of the Social Security Act in 1990, beneficiaries of all benefit schemes (except the WCS and private insurance) were required to receive care in public hospitals, with limited reimbursements obtainable for civil servants for private hospital inpatient care. Under the WCS and private insurance, beneficiaries are free to choose either public or private hospitals to receive care. At that time, the role of private hospitals was limited to providing care to the population covered by these two schemes and those few who could afford higher fees in private hospitals.

The SSS opened up an opportunity for private hospitals to play an increasing role in the provision of care. The extent to which private hospitals are utilized depends on the incentive mechanisms and conditions governing the hospitals' entrance into the scheme and their operation, as well as the level of choice of providers and ease of access to the services.

6.5.1   Objectives and administration

The main objectives of the SSS are to reduce inequity in access to health care of different population groups, and to provide security to the insured despite unpredictable fluctuations in health care expenditures. The scheme is based on risk-sharing principles in providing access to health services to employees of all types of business establishments when they become ill, regardless of income or economic and social status. At present the scheme is confined to employees in the formal sector since they are the most manageable group.

The SSS was established and implemented under the provisions of the Social Security Act of 1990. It is operated by the Social Security Office (SSO) under the Ministry of Labor and Social Welfare. The SSO administers the Social Security Fund from which insured persons receive benefits under the Act. The fund receives contributions from three parties: the employers, the employees, and the government, each paying 1.5 per cent of the employee's wages, to a maximum limit of wages of 500 baht per day or 15 000 baht per month. Hence the contributions have a regressive structure, with lower-wage employees paying a higher percentage of their wages than higher-income employees.

The 1.5 per cent contribution rate by each party is allocated to various benefits as follows: 0.88 per cent for illness benefits, 0.12 per cent for maternity benefits, 0.44 per cent for disability benefits, and 0.06 per cent for death benefits. Total contributions averaged 464 million baht per month in 1991 and increased each year to over 1 billion baht per month in 1995.

With continued increases in revenue and low rates of utilization of benefits between 1991 and 1994, the total revenue of the Social Security Fund amounted to over 31.5 billion baht, while expenditures were only 9.2 billion baht, yielding a surplus of more than 22 billion baht by 1995. Each year the unused funds have been invested in banks and government enterprises rather than being used to reduce premiums or expand benefits.

The SSO also administers the WCS, an insurance scheme complementary to the SSS. The WCS compensates work-related illnesses and injuries, disability, and death.

6.5.2 Coverage: benefits and population

At present, the 1990 Social Security Act extends comprehensive coverage to nonwork-related illnesses, disability, and death, as well as maternity benefits. It will be extended to include old-age pensions and family allowances in the second stage, probably by 1998, and unemployment benefits when appropriate. However, contributions will have to increase. The Act requires that private employees in all establishments with 20 or more employees be covered starting in March 1991 and, in September 1993, it was extended to establishments with 10 or more employees. However, Article 55 of the Act states that employers already providing any benefit better than that offered by the SSS do not have to join the scheme for that particular type of benefit and the contributions to the fund are reduced accordingly. This article has created an administrative burden to the fund due to employees receiving different benefits from their employers. Most of the exemptions are for strong companies, resulting in only weaker ones joining the Social Security Fund. If these firms do not maintain their contributions, the fund could become financially unstable.

In September 1994, benefits were extended to those insured on a voluntary basis. Those include private enterprises with fewer than 10 employees, the self-employed — such as farmers and traders — and other uninsured groups. However, arguments have been raised regarding "selection bias", a weakness connected with voluntary health insurance schemes. High-risk individuals and those with chronic illness who anticipate net benefits from their contributions will join the scheme, while low-risk individuals will not, causing a heavy financial burden on the scheme. There is also a problem, still unresolved, about the third party's contribution. In addition, calculation of contributions from the self-employed and farmers may incur substantial administrative costs to the scheme. It has sometimes been argued that a voluntary health insurance scheme such as the health card program would be a more appropriate form of coverage for the self-employed.

As of October 1995, 5.25 million workers in 72 500 establishments were insured under the SSS. This number of workers represents about 15 per cent of the labor force, 55 per cent of private sector employees, and 8.8 per cent of the population.

Illness benefits consist of general and specialized services, outpatient services, hospital care, pharmaceutical expenses, ambulance costs, and other necessary expenses. Certain conditions and services are not covered by the scheme, such as drug addiction, hospitalization for over 180 days, cosmetic services, infertility, hemodialysis, psychogenic illness, organ transplantation, dental services, and glasses and lenses.

In addition to free health care provided to the insured at the registered hospitals, there are cash benefits to compensate the insured on sick leave, maternity leave, and disability: at 50 per cent of wages, up to 90 days each time with a maximum of 180 days per year for illness, up to 90 days with a maximum of two confinements for maternity, and for the duration of a disability.

6.5.3 Health care providers and provider payment methods

Health care providers under the SSS consist of both public and private facilities. Public facilities include provincial and community hospitals, community health posts under the MOPH, university hospitals, Bangkok Metropolitan Administration hospitals, state enterprises hospitals, and hospitals belonging to the Ministry of Defense. Private facilities consist of general and special hospitals, polyclinics (providing many outpatient specialty services), and clinics (one physician).

Hospitals can enter the SSS as main contractors with licenses issued by the SSO, upon meeting the hospital standards set out by the Medical Committee. These standards include provision of general medical care, accident and emergency care, outpatient care, inpatient care, intensive care, surgical care, and anesthesiological, radiological, pathological, medical registration, and pharmaceutical practice standards. In broad terms, the hospitals must have at least 100 beds, a good referral system, and be well equipped, with all types of necessary facilities. The main contractor may contract with hospitals providing lower levels of care, called subcontractors, and those providing higher levels of care, called supracontractors.

From 1991 to 1996, the number of main contractors under the SSS increased from 137 to 199. While the number of public hospitals increased slightly, from 117 to 124, the number of private hospitals has expanded significantly, from 18 in 1991 to 73 in 1996. In the first year of implementation, very few private hospitals joined the scheme, for fear of making a loss, given the fixed capitation payment, while public hospitals under the MOPH were required to provide care to the insured under the scheme. Low utilization rates in the first year generated profits for most providers in the SSS, which provided incentives for others to participate. After the second year of the scheme's operation, more and more private hospitals entered as main contractors, and an increasing number of the insured registered with private hospitals.

The rapid growth in the number of private hospitals joining the SSS has resulted from both demand and supply factors. On the supply side, there was an expansion in the number of private hospitals in Bangkok and nearby provinces; profit incentives motivated them to join the scheme. On the demand side, there was increased utilization by the insured as their numbers grew and they were better informed about their eligibility for benefits.

Hospitals contracted under the SSS are paid a capitation fee of 700 baht per insured person registered with the hospital, regardless of actual utilization. Capitation was chosen as a provider payment method over fee-for-service, which is used in the WCS. This choice was made to prevent cost escalation and for simplicity of administration, as well as for the security of the fund. The 700 baht capitation rate is calculated on the basis of an average of three outpatient visits per year at 150 baht per visit and 0.5 inpatient days per year at 500 baht per day. This rate was used from 1990 until the end of 1995. Beginning in 1996, the capitation payment will increase to 800 baht per insured person.

The capitation payment method helps contain costs due to a more rational use of diagnostic procedures, drugs, and treatments than the fee-for-service method. Administrative costs of the scheme are also low, since there is no need for claim screening as in the case of fee-for-service. Moreover, capitation creates incentives for providers to compete to obtain a larger market share of the insured and, if a good quality control mechanism exists, better quality of care can be achieved as a result of the competition.

Capitation has some disadvantages, however, such as inconvenience for users, who have to receive care only from the registered hospital and a tendency for hospitals to limit services or to lower quality in order to control costs. Some measures have been undertaken by the SSO to correct these disadvantages. To increase accessibility of services and improve efficiency in health care delivery, the SSO has encouraged the formation of a provider network whereby small hospitals unable to provide certain services can refer their patients to the main contractor in the network.

An example of the development of a network of primary health care facilities is a pilot project of Nopparat Rajathanee Hospital from June to December 1993. The project consisted of private clinics and polyclinics attached to a public general hospital in Bangkok. At the start of the project, 38 health care facilities (28 private) formed a network of public–private facilities providing outpatient care for the insured registered with Nopparat Rajathanee Hospital. By the end of the project, there were 50 health facilities participating, 40 of which were private. The total utilization rate for the network increased during project implementation from 32.3 to 133.9 visits per 1000 insured persons per month, while it declined for public hospitals. Moreover, the project has caused an increase of 69 per cent in the number of insured persons registered at Nopparat Rajathanee Hospital. A database of all outpatient visits to the whole network was established, enabling the monitoring of the quality of care of each health care facility and the disease pattern of the insured.

Under normal circumstances, the insured has to go to the hospital where he or she has registered to receive health care. However, in an emergency, the insured can receive care at any hospital and seek reimbursement from the Social Security Fund but has to inform the SSO and be transferred to the registered hospital within 3 days. This arrangement for partial reimbursement of emergency treatment was made after many incidents of refusal by noncontracted hospitals to treat accident victims.

To extend the range of services available to the insured, the Social Security Fund makes additional payments to the contracted hospitals for services with high costs of treatment (hemodialysis, chemotherapy, open heart surgery, brain surgery) and services with high rates of utilization.

6.6   HEALTH SERVICE UTILIZATION UNDER THE SOCIAL SECURITY SCHEME

6.6.1   Utilization rates and patterns

Utilization of benefits from the SSS was very low at the beginning but increased from 0.6 million cases in 1991 to 3.44 million cases in 1995. During this time, benefit payments increased from 19 per cent of the contributions in 1991 to 34 per cent. Illness benefits have the highest utilization, averaging 411 300 cases per month in 1995, while that of maternity was 17 600 cases. Death and disability benefits have the lowest utilization rates.

For illness benefits, the average utilization was initially very low. The average number of outpatient visits expanded fivefold, from 81 000 per month in 1991 to 400 000 per month in 1995. The number of inpatient cases almost tripled, from 4000 per month to almost 12 000 between 1991 and 1994. In terms of utilization, Table 6.4 indicates that the outpatient use rate increased from 0.71 to 1.33 visits per insured person per year between 1992 and 1995, while the per capita inpatient use rate for insured workers remained unchanged.

Table 6.4 also shows utilization by type of provider. Outpatient utilization in public facilities increased by 78 per cent while the increase in private facilities was 169 per cent. The use of inpatient care declined over 16 per cent in public facilities but increased nearly 50 per cent in private facilities. Private hospitals accounted for 64 per cent of total outpatient visits and 60 per cent of inpatient admissions in 1995. This compares to their share of 54 per cent for outpatient utilization and 46 per cent for inpatient admissions in 1992.

6.6.2   Factors affecting utilization and choice of providers

The low utilization rate at the beginning of the SSS was due mainly to a number of conditions limiting its use. During the first year of operation, employers chose providers for their employees. This was because the information system of the SSO was not ready, and matching employees' choices with the hospitals was difficult. Surveys indicated that the employers tended to choose hospitals on the basis of proximity to the workplace, good medical services, and past relationship with hospitals under the WCS. Consequently, there was a problem of accessibility to the registered hospitals since employees' residences were not necessarily close to the hospitals. Moreover, many employees, such as construction workers and sales representatives, tend to be very mobile. This problem was alleviated when employees were able gradually to choose their own providers from 1992 onward. By the end of 1996, all insured workers will be able to choose their own registered hospital.

Other factors contributing to the initial low utilization rate were the lack of understanding on the part of the insured about the benefits that they were entitled to

Table 6.4. Utilization of Medical Services by Those Insured through the Social Security Scheme, 1992 and 1995.

	1992			1995[a]			Change, 1992–95
	Public	Private and others	Total	Public	Private and others	Total	
Number of health facilities for Social Security enrollees	116	29	145	110	61	171	+18%
Number of insured workers registered (thousands)	1703	1052	2755	1417	1941	3358	+22%
Outpatient visits (thousands)	899	1062	1961	1602	2853	4455	+127%
Inpatient admissions (thousands)	49	42	91	41	62	103	+13%
Average length of stay (days)	6.7	3.0	5.0	5.5	3.9	4.5	−10%
Outpatient visits per insured person per year	0.53	1.01	0.71	1.13	1.47	1.33	+87%
Inpatient use rate per insured person per year	0.03	0.04	0.03	0.03	0.03	0.03	0%

[a]Annualized, based on January–June 1995 data.
Source: Social Security Office, Bangkok, Thailand, 1995.

receive from the SSS and the procedures and conditions involved in the utilization of services at the registered hospitals; the SSO was not ready to issue membership cards to the insured to facilitate utilization of services from providers; and providers were ill prepared in terms of space, equipment, and personnel to provide services to the insured.

As discussed above, measures were employed to remedy the disadvantages of capitation payment to providers. These included encouraging provider networks and partial reimbursement of emergency treatments, as well as additional payments to providers for services with high costs of treatment and high rates of utilization. Cases of complaints were inspected, perhaps increasing the rate of utilization. The insured were given more convenient access to health care and providers were more willing to offer a wider range of services to the insured. The insured are now able to choose their own providers each year, which could improve the quality of services and their satisfaction with them.

Nonthaburi, located close to Bangkok, is the pilot province where, as of 1992, the insured can choose their own providers. A case study (Patichon, 1995) of the behavior of the insured in this province was carried out from 1991 to 1993. During those years, the number of hospitals contracted with the SSO to serve the insured in Nonthaburi increased from two public hospitals in 1991 to 15 public and four private hospitals in 1992, and 23 public and 25 private hospitals in 1993. At the same time, the number of insured people in the province increased from 31 255 in 1991 to 56 446 in 1992 (a 44.6 per cent increase) and 56 548 in 1993. In 1991, all the insured had to register with one of the two public hospitals, the choice of which was made by their employers.

The study found that very few of the insured changed providers (8 per cent in 1992 and 10 per cent in 1993). This was explained by the fact that most of the insured lacked experience in receiving care and had no information about the quality of services of available providers. Moreover, the process involved in changing providers was still rather complicated and time-consuming. It was also found that the location of the hospital was another important factor explaining the small change, since 48 per cent of the insured chose providers located in the province and the two contracted public hospitals were within the province, while most additional providers were located outside.

There is an increasing tendency for the insured to select private providers, due, in part, to the increasing number of private providers enrolled and available for members' selection under the scheme. The increase is gradual, however: the choice of a private provider by the insured increased from 2 per cent in 1992 to 4.4 per cent in 1993. The change is incremental because very few insured members change providers and when they initially enrolled in the scheme the number of private providers available was small. By contrast, for hospital care most of the insured chose the private hospital in the province: of 300 insured workers interviewed, the number of those who chose a private hospital rather than a public hospital increased from 12 per cent in 1992 to 28 per cent in 1993.

6.6.3   Changes in health-seeking behavior

A study of health-seeking behavior of the insured working in Samut Prakan province in 1992 (Tangcharoensathien *et al.*, 1993) revealed that the pattern of health service utilization has not changed significantly since the implementation of the SSS. Before the SSS, self-prescribed drugs were the dominant means of care for those with minor illness, followed by private clinics and services in the medical room at the workplace. Among those who sought care at hospitals, over 50 per cent went to private hospitals. The survey conducted in 1992 found that, although the pattern of care-seeking is similar to that before the SSS, the relative importance in terms of proportion of use has changed; for example, the percentage of illness episodes treated with self-prescribed drugs declined to 28 per cent for outpatients and to 16 per cent for private clinics. Hospital visits increased from 6 per cent to 25 per cent and the market share of private hospitals increased to over 90 per cent.

Before the SSS, for cases of severe illness, 75 per cent went to hospitals and 22 per cent went to clinics but, after the scheme had been implemented for 1 year, 80 per cent of inpatient cases went to hospitals and only 8 per cent went to clinics.

Similarly, a comparison of health care-seeking behavior in Nonthaburi before the SSS and by members of the scheme in 1992 and 1993 (Patichon, 1995) has indicated a reduction in the proportion of the ill who sought no treatment and those who used self-prescribed drugs and services of the medical room at the workplace. On the other hand, the use of hospital care increased significantly, with registered public hospitals providing more services than registered private hospitals. For nonmembers of the scheme, however, there was no change in the use of private hospitals and self-prescribed drugs, but an increased use of private clinics instead of medical services at the workplace.

In contrast to the changes under the SSS, medical care for those involved in car accidents under the Protection of Motor Vehicle Accident Victims Act of 1992 has been provided mostly in public hospitals. One explanation for this is that the average expenditure for the care of car accident patients in a private hospital is about eight times higher than in a public hospital (Nittayaramphong *et al.*, 1995).

6.7   THE SOCIAL SECURITY SCHEME AND PRIVATE HEALTH SECTOR GROWTH

Private providers have been gaining an increasing share of the insured under the SSS. Table 6.5 suggests that despite fewer contracted facilities the market share of private hospitals has continued to rise at the expense of public hospitals, particularly the MOPH hospitals. The formation of a provider network is a strategy used to expand the market share, by increasing accessibility to medical services. As utilization rates expand, hospitals must find ways to compete for the insured, so that they can cope with rising costs and maintain profits. The larger the number of private hospitals joining the scheme, the stronger is their ability to attract customers.

In choosing their location, many new private hospitals have selected large industrial areas with great potential for a large number of insured employees to register with them. Another strategy of competing with other private hospitals is to use the brand names of well-established hospitals when branching out to new communities. The brand-name marketing strategy is used by many well-known hospitals, such as Bamrungrad, Samiteivej, Phyathai, and Bangkok Hospitals.

Table 6.5. Number of Public and Private Health Facilities and Percentage of Market Share under the Social Security Scheme.

Health facilities	1991		1993		1995	
	Number	% Market share	Number	% Market share	Number	% Market share
Public health facilities	117	50.2	117	43.0	123	33.8
Ministry of Defense	12	7.1	13	3.8	14	2.1
Ministry of Interior	5	6.1	5	3.2	5	2.1
Ministry of Public Health	94	30.4	93	29.6	98	24.9
Ministry of University Affairs	6	6.6	6	6.4	6	4.7
Private health facilities	18	43.9	37	52.4	63	63.2
Others	2	5.9	2	4.6	3	3.0
Total	137	100.0	156	100.0	189	100.0

Source: Social Security Office, Bangkok, Thailand, 1995.

Private hospitals also compete on the basis of quality of services, such as attentive and courteous care, short waiting time, clean and attractively decorated rooms, fine food, computerization of medical records, office automation, wide-ranging personal services, and parking spaces. In addition, many private hospitals provide special services in their centers for specialized treatments. These centers are often equipped with the latest high-cost medical technology and are staffed by well-known specialists recruited from public hospitals. Some other private hospitals attempt to attract the insured by offering additional features to their social security campaign, such as preventive medical programs and mobile clinics.

More and more urban people already use private hospitals, in spite of their higher prices, because they offer greater convenience and accessibility, shorter waiting time, and new medical equipment and facilities. The trend is also for employees insured under the SSS to turn more to private providers to enjoy such conveniences, especially in terms of location. Since it is highly unlikely that public hospitals will increase in number, it is the private hospitals that will take up the increase in the insured as benefits of the SSS expand to cover other population groups in the future. There is, therefore, much room for further private sector growth in providing health care under insurance schemes in Thailand. Competition among private providers could bring about not only increased efficiency in containing costs, but also better quality of services, as the insured are better informed about the benefits they are entitled to receive under the scheme and the choices of services available to them.

6.8   CONCLUSION

The rapid expansion of private hospitals in Thailand in the past decade has been due to rising income, demographic changes, increased education, and the government's investment and promotional measures. Bangkok has benefited most from the private sector growth in health care. A large number of new hospitals are located in the capital or nearby provinces, while other regions have gained fewer new private hospitals and beds.

Since this pattern of growth of the private sector has been ongoing for some time, it can be anticipated that the trend will continue in the future. Most of the new private hospitals will still be in Bangkok and the surrounding areas. It is estimated that the number of private hospital beds in Bangkok between 1994 and 1997 will increase by 6000. These trends will exacerbate the unevenness in the distribution of private hospitals in the country.

Given these estimates and the fact that the bed occupancy rate in private hospitals is only 58 per cent compared with 99 per cent in public hospitals (Nittayaramphong and Tangcharoensathien, 1994), it is clear that there is much room for private hospitals to expand in other provinces. The high public occupancy rates in Bangkok imply a supply shortage. In fact, many large hospitals have started to branch out into the provinces to provide care under the SSS, which has generated increasing demand for hospital care among the employed.

The SSS has been in effect in Thailand for 5 years. It has provided about 5 million workers, almost 9 per cent of the population, with four types of benefits, including nonwork-related illness, disability, maternity, and death benefits. During this time, significant increases in rates of utilization and changes in patterns of service utilization by the insured employees have occurred. The role of private providers in the scheme has increased as well. A clear trend among the insured is a reduction in self-prescribed drugs and visits to private clinics, while hospital visits increased substantially in both public and private sectors. The shift of SSS beneficiaries to private providers raises interesting policy questions for the government. Should it continue to fund public hospitals that do not compare well? Should the government withdraw its financial support to public hospitals if they cannot attract SSS enrollees? Private providers have gained more than 50 per cent of the market share of the insured employees, and incentives exist to continue competing for further expansion. Various nonprice strategies have been used to attract customers. What is still lacking in the system is a quality control mechanism to ensure that profit motives and competition to gain market share will not lead to worsening quality of services.

Thailand is now at the crossroads for health care reform. On one hand, health care expenditure is rising faster than general economic growth. On the other hand, there is a policy to expand insurance coverage to the entire population, which could generate further expenditure increases. There are many options to consider in order to achieve the objectives of equity and efficiency in health financing and health delivery systems while maintaining good-quality services. In all of these options, the private sector has an important role to play both as a source of financing and as a provider of services.

REFERENCES

Chunharas, S., Kittidilokkul, S. (1992). *Medical Personnel: Transfers between the Public and Private Sectors*. Paper presented at the Seminar on the Role of the Private Sector in the Thai Health Sector, Bangkok.

Myers, C., Mongkolsmai, D., Causino, N. (1985). *Financing Health Services and Medical Care in Thailand*. Report prepared for USAID, Bangkok.

Nittayaramphong, S., Tangcharoensathien, V. (1994). Thailand: private health care out of control? *Health Policy and Planning*, **9**(1), 31–40.

Nittayaramphong, S., Saelim, S., Kaugwallert, R. (1995). *A Study of Health Service Provision to Motor Vehicle Accident Victims under Act B.E. 2535*. Bangkok: Office of Health Insurance and the Bureau of Health Policy and Planning, Ministry of Public Health (in Thai).

Patichon, P. (1995). *Choice of Provider and Utilization of Medical Services among Insured Persons under the Social Security Scheme in Nonthaburi*. MA Thesis, Faculty of Economics, Thammasat University, Bangkok (in Thai).

Social Security Office. (1995). Unpublished data, Bangkok.

Tangcharoensathien, V., Kamonratanakul, P., Supachutikul, A. (1993). *Health-Seeking Behavior of Insured Workers in Samut Prakan in 1992*. Health Insurance Monograph Series No. 61. Bangkok: Office of Health Policy and Planning, Ministry of Public Health (in Thai).

Part III
Supply-Side Issues and Lessons

7

Supply-Side Approaches to Optimizing Private Health Sector Growth

PETER BERMAN

Associate Professor, Harvard School of Public Health

7.1 INTRODUCTION

It is widely agreed that a health care system left to function according to market forces alone will not result in a socially optimal quantity or quality of health care or cost (Hsiao, 1995). Health care markets suffer from significant deviations from the pure competitive model proposed in economics, and these deviations can result in significant losses of social welfare.[1] Some health care services and the distribution of health benefits also have merit characteristics that call for action beyond what the market might provide. As a result, extensive social intervention in the health care market is justified in relation to the financing and provision of health care generally, and to its distribution in the population.

In many developing countries, a commitment to such social intervention was made through constitutional guarantees of the rights of access to health care for all. Countries invested in government-owned and government-run systems of hospitals, clinics, medical training and research institutions, and production facilities for health care inputs (such as drugs) as their primary approach to fulfilling such guarantees. Services provided by these institutions were usually available at little or no direct cost to the beneficiaries.

Most governments have not, by themselves, provided health care services in public institutions at a level sufficient to meet the population's demands. The result — again nearly universal in the developing world — is that private health care expenditure on services provided by private health care practitioners and facilities usually accounts for a large share, and often for the majority, of total spending. Private providers usually account for a significant share of total service output and, for major parts of

---

[1] See also Chapter 2 by Rosenthal and Newbrander and Chapter 4 by Jeffers.

Private Health Sector Growth in Asia: Issues and Implications. Edited by W. Newbrander.
© 1997 John Wiley & Sons, Ltd.

the health care system, such as ambulatory treatment of illness, they may account for the largest share.

In Asia, there is a widespread perception that private health care provision is growing rapidly. It is often implied that such growth may be excessive, for instance, that it will greatly exceed population or income growth. Since reliable data on the size and composition of private health care provision are lacking in many countries and are even less available in time series, it is hard to verify this perception. For the more visible changes, such as increases in large private hospitals, such trends may, however, be self-evident.

These changes are widely perceived as problems that require a policy response. This chapter will address these issues in terms of four questions. First, what are some of the problems associated with private health care provision and its growth that may require a policy response? Conversely, what might be some of the opportunities for advancing social goals afforded by an expanding private sector? Second, what can be done to increase positive outcomes and reduce the problems through government action, specifically those interventions that operate on the supply side of the market? Third, what are some recent Asian experiences in these areas that may be relevant to other countries in Asia? Fourth, what practical constraints to intervention exist?

7.2   PRIVATE SECTOR GROWTH

This chapter deals almost exclusively with issues related to private *provision* of health care, in contrast to private *financing* (for example, the growth of private household spending or private insurance development). Private financing raises many issues beyond the scope of the discussion presented in this chapter.

What distinguishes private sector from public sector health care? Bennett (1992) defines private sector health care as those parts of the health care system not under the direct control of the government. One obvious dimension is ownership. But the concept of control implies more. It suggests that private health care can function according to a different set of objectives and norms. It reflects the fact that private health care providers may seek profits, choose which services to provide, and determine their own levels of quality, mix of inputs, and costs. These freedoms are seen by many to have the potential for negative social outcomes in the form of high-cost, low-quality, and exploitative behavior. On the positive side, it is clear that private providers can significantly augment the total quantity of health care available. For example, these same freedoms can also be a source of innovation in both the for-profit and not-for-profit private health care sectors. They may result in more efficient, higher-quality services and greater patient satisfaction.

Countries are increasingly looking to the experiences of other nations in their search for appropriate health sector policies. With regard to the role of private health care provision in national health systems, the experience of the Organization for Economic Cooperation and Development (OECD) member countries does not indicate either universally positive or negative outcomes. Canada and Sweden are countries with similar levels of health spending as a percentage of income. Both are regarded as having highly successful health care systems. In Canada, most primary care providers are private practitioners paid on the basis of fee-for-service (OECD, 1995). In Sweden, they are paid mostly by salary from local government authorities. If we look at health systems in other OECD countries (including some of the systems most successful in improving access and health, controlling costs, and assuring client satisfaction), we find significant variability in ownership of both primary care and hospital facilities. In other words, the experience of industrialized countries suggests that it is possible to organize a health care system in such a way that both public and privately owned providers can contribute to efficient and equitable health care. Ownership seems not to be a significant determinant when modified by appropriate structuring of the health care market in terms of financing, service delivery, and demand.

This does not mean that, under other conditions, ownership does not matter, nor does it signify that it should not be a matter of concern in Asia. There are other examples in the OECD, such as the USA, of very costly health care systems with almost entirely private provision (including a sizable nonprofit sector) and significant private financing. Rather, it suggests that we should look carefully at what type of problems growing private health care provision might cause, and what are the means for controlling those problems. Direct control, for which governments' main tools have been ownership and administrative determination of inputs and functioning, is not the only type of control that is possible.

7.2.1 Problems

There are at least five major concerns about the effects of private health care provision from the perspective of national health policy goals and objectives. These are:

1. Private providers respond to the population's willingness to pay for health care. As a result, they will serve those groups in the population most willing to pay, such as affluent urban residents. The result will be increased inequity in access and use of health care.
2. Because of lower willingness to pay, private providers will undersupply socially desirable services, such as immunizations and personal preventive care. This will worsen allocative efficiency in the health sector.
3. Driven by the profit motive, and because they have significant control over demand, private providers will take advantage of patients by supplying more health care than is required. This is inefficient and may result in health-impairing actions.
4. Private providers can also take advantage of patients by providing low-quality health care, which may result in health and welfare losses.
5. Private health care will draw scarce human and physical resources away from public sector needs. This will also result in allocative inefficiency, through underprovision of services.

Each of these concerns can be related to specific market failures or insufficient response to socially desirable objectives. In (1) above, the issue is one of social merit. To the extent that societies seek to assure health care to groups less able to pay (on grounds such as poverty, location, and gender), private providers responding to market demand will, left on their own, not provide the socially desired level of services. If these underserved groups are also the least healthy, as they often are, this bias in provision will also result in lower health gains from a given level of health expenditure.

In (2) and (5), the question is related to well-known market failures from the existence of social benefits greater than individual benefits from certain interventions. Such externalities and the possibility of individuals benefiting as "free riders" from the actions of others result in insufficient demand by consumers for certain interventions. Responding to that demand, private providers will provide less than the socially desirable quantity of care. Indirectly, they can have a similar effect at the sectoral level by making it difficult for government to finance and procure essential inputs like staff and supplies.

In (3) and (4), the negative effects are related to the inequality of information between patient and provider. Much of the demand for health care is decided by the provider on behalf of the patient. The provider is also the authority, in the eyes of the patient, on what is needed. The provider can benefit personally from providing both a greater quantity or sophistication of service than may be objectively needed by the patient and the provider can also subtly reduce the quality of service provided without the patient's knowledge. Such conflicts of interest, when the provider acts as an agent for the patient yet has a financial interest different from that of just benefiting the patient, can lead to high-cost and poor-quality services.

The presence of insurance, nearly universal in industrialized countries, has a significant effect on these problems, but does not eliminate them. Indeed, it may make some of them worse. Insurance can greatly reduce the differences in willingness to pay in a population, reducing in importance point (1) above. However, this may exacerbate the problems described in (3), especially when the insurer pays providers for any service provided, as they did for many years in the USA. This introduces a third party with interests and responsibilities into the patient–provider relationship. When the insurer also has strong profit motivations, it may introduce additional pressures to reduce quantity or quality of service, or it may be able to provide a professional counterbalance to the provider's inclinations in that regard.

Is the profit motive the main problem here? Research in the USA, where most hospitals are not-for-profit entities, suggests that even nonprofits have incentives to behave in ways that are often similar to for-profits. It has been noted that, while nonprofits may devote more resources to social objectives, such as medical training and care for the indigent, they also accumulate financial surpluses, which can be appropriated by managers in various ways, including higher salaries. This has led some to question whether the social benefits are worth the significant tax concessions such entities receive.

It is also important to note that government is not without its failures. Bureaucratic management of diverse and dispersed health care facilities has often resulted in disappointing outcomes in countries at all levels of income. The internal market reforms of the UK (such as autonomy for public sector hospitals and greater financial authority for salaried general practitioners) are a response to perceived shortcomings of public management. The shortcomings of public sector health services in developing countries, including resource imbalances, low productivity, and poor quality, are well known.

7.2.2   Opportunities

The growth of private health care certainly represents a response to increasing demands of the population, including both the quantity of health care desired as well as preferences about the way in which it is provided. There is widespread evidence that private ambulatory providers, including both formally qualified and informal providers of various types, are used by people at all income levels, including those of low income.[2] They are also used extensively in the treatment of diseases of public health importance, such as diarrhea, respiratory infections, tuberculosis, sexually transmitted diseases (STDs), malaria, and others. Some types of private health care providers may be even more prevalent in rural areas than government services.

In lower-income countries, health care providers who are numerous, distributed to underserved areas, and acceptable and accessible to the poor may indeed offer an opportunity to expand access to and coverage of essential basic services. While the quality of training received and care offered by these providers may be low, one should not ignore such a resource in environments of significant resource scarcity. What can these providers contribute to achieving urgent public health goals?

The development of higher-level private facilities, such as medium-sized and large hospitals, may also offer opportunities for advancing public sector health goals. Private providers can substitute for costly publicly provided services that may be of low priority. They can replace government investments in ancillary facilities and services, such as diagnostic facilities and support services in hospitals. In urban areas, private ambulatory care providers may be able to function as substitutes for government-financed health centers and dispensaries.

7.2.3   Diagnosis of the situation

The problems and opportunities related to the private health sector in Asia cannot be properly assessed without a good understanding of the structure of the national and local health care systems within which private health care functions. Asian countries vary dramatically in their levels of income, education, urbanization, formal sector employment, and health care resources. These factors are important determinants of the specific types of problems they might encounter with private health care.

In addition to these indicators of national conditions, specific knowledge about the organization of health care provision is needed. Most countries in the region lack adequate information about the numbers and types of private health care

---

[2]See chapters 6, 8, 9, and 11 in this volume, on Thailand, India, the Philippines, and Indonesia, respectively.

practitioners and facilities, their location, who they serve, and what type of services they provide. There are also specific institutional conditions that are not well described or understood. These conditions relate to the structure of specific facilities such as hospitals, clinics, and diagnostic units and the functional and commercial relationships between them. For example, in India and the Philippines, rapid growth of small private hospitals has been reported (Bhat, 1993b; Griffin *et al.*, 1994). What are these facilities, often having 10 beds or less? What services do they provide? What is their relationship to physicians' outpatient practices and to higher-level hospitals? Alternatively, what are the relationships between physicians' practices, pharmacies, and free-standing diagnostic facilities?

A unique aspect of private health care in many Asian countries is the presence of private practitioners who are not part of the usual cosmopolitan health care systems. This refers not only to traditional practitioners, but to the "eclectic, less than fully qualified" providers, who are particularly prevalent in South Asia. In India, one recent study estimated that more than 1 million of such providers are active, a rate of more than 1 per 1000 population — not including the qualified practitioners of different systems of medicine (Rohde and Vishwanathan, 1995). These providers are also present in other countries and include informal drug sellers, partially qualified paramedics in private practice, and others. Such providers are often uncounted and unregulated, yet they provide services that may be indistinguishable for much of the population from those of qualified providers. (The same Indian study found that 83 per cent of providers called "doctor" by rural women were not fully qualified.) These providers are widespread and account for a high proportion of total coverage with personal health care services. At present, we understand little about how these providers work, what they do, whom they reach, and what their effect on the overall health care market is.

Another important dimension of private health care in Asia is the presence of insurance, as summarized in Table 7.1. In most countries of the region, social health insurance is available for a small portion of the population, usually including formal sector workers and civil servants. Private health insurance, including employers' direct financing of health care, is also present mainly for the better-off population in urban areas. However, this group may account for a disproportionate share of those having contact with private health care providers. This may be especially true if social insurance pays for treatment by private providers, as it does in Thailand, the Philippines, Indonesia, and Korea.

As is well known, the presence of insurance can substantially affect the behavior of both providers and users of health care. With insurance, price plays less of a role in a patient's decision to seek care. Providers (both physicians and hospitals) may also feel justified in augmenting services since the patient will not bear the burden of payment. Insurers can also become active managers of health care. How significant is insurance in the dynamics of private sector development in different countries? What parts of the private health sector are most affected?

In many Asian countries, there exists a wide range of informal linkages between public and private health care practice. Some examples of this follow. First, publicly employed physicians and paramedics in many countries may be entitled to engage in private practice after official hours. Second, in some countries, private physicians

Table 7.1. Health Insurance Coverage in Selected Asian Countries.

Country	Social health insurance coverage (% of population)	Private health insurance coverage (% of population)
Taiwan[a]	100	0
Thailand[b]	27	2
Papua New Guinea[c]	0	< 1
Vietnam[d]	38	< 1
India[e]	3	< 1
Korea[f]	100	< 1
Indonesia	17[g]	1[h]
China[i]	19	< 1
Philippines[j]	42	NA
Sri Lanka[k]	0	1.5

Sources: [a]1995 data from Department of Health, the Executive Yuan, People's Republic of China, 1995; [b]Smutharaks (1993); [c]1992 data from Thomason (1992); [d]Solon et al. (1995); [e]1991 figures adapted from World Bank (1995); [f]Yang, Chapter 5; [g]Solon et al. (1995); [h]1989 data from Paqueo and Lieberman (1992); [i]National Health Survey (1993); [j]1991 data from Patao and Jeffers (1994); [k]Ravi Rannan-Eliya, conversation with author, Cambridge, MA, 1996. NA, not available.

may be able to admit and treat patients privately in public hospitals, receiving private fees for themselves and having patients pay highly subsidized charges (or no charges) for clinical facilities, nursing, diagnostic, and other support services. Third, despite low or no charges for services in public facilities, household surveys often report much higher out-of-pocket payments from patients for use of government health centers and hospitals. Such unofficial charges may reflect an informal fee-for-service payment system to physicians and nurses in the government health facility that co-exists with the official fee-for-service payment system of the public facility. For all these examples, we could ask about effects on public and private health care provision and on the costs, quality, equity, and effectiveness of the health services overall.

The preceding examples all point to the need to understand better the structure and dynamics of the health care market in Asian countries, with special attention to the institutional aspects of the supply side of the market.

7.2.4 Specific developments

Recent studies have highlighted a number of developments regarding private sector growth in Asia. These have often been accompanied by concerns about the impact of these developments on national health care systems.

7.2.4.1 Rapid growth of sophisticated urban-based private hospitals. It is widely perceived that privately owned secondary and tertiary hospitals are growing rapidly in some countries. This is seen as causing problems related to rapidly rising costs, such as increased—and possibly unnecessary use of—sophisticated medical technology. This issue has been noted in Thailand, where it is seen as placing unsustainable financial pressures on the newly expanded national health insurance program (Nittayaramphong and Tangcharoensathien, 1994). Growth in this sector may have significant effects on total national health spending, on the costs of specific health care services, and even on the costs of public sector provision, through bidding up the wages and prices of health care inputs.

7.2.4.2 Rapid growth of small inpatient facilities. The proliferation of small inpatient facilities has been noted in the Philippines (Griffin *et al.*, 1994), and India (Bhat, 1993b). In the Philippines, it has been diagnosed as a market response to new financing opportunities from the Medicare health insurance program. In India, these facilities, known as nursing homes, probably account for a large share of private inpatient facilities and beds. Such facilities may allow private physicians to capture significant earnings for care of patients, while providing only a modest range of services of limited quality. These facilities, while more affordable than the larger hospitals, may not be capable of providing adequate services for inpatient care. Which sections of the population they serve, and at what cost, is unclear.

7.2.4.3 High levels of use of ambulatory care from less than fully qualified providers. There is broad concern about the quality of care and cost of private ambulatory treatment of different types. One can identify at least the following:

- Direct diagnosis, prescribing, and dispensing by pharmacists and other drug sellers. In much of Asia, officially controlled pharmaceuticals are widely available from a variety of sources, without proper prescriptions and controls. This can be associated with inappropriate prescribing, and poor counseling and patient follow-up
- Unregulated practice by less than fully qualified practitioners. As noted above, in some countries, particularly those of South Asia, unqualified practice is extremely widespread and accounts for the majority of ambulatory health care contacts
- Unregulated practice by new forms of diagnostic facilities. Private, free-standing diagnostic facilities providing radiology (X-ray, ultrasonography, computed tomography [CT] scans) and laboratory services are proliferating. To what extent do these facilities become primary care centers in practice?
- Expanded availability of new health commodities such as herbal medicines and tonics.

As noted earlier, this pattern of development in Asian health care systems presents both problems and opportunities. Poor-quality care by unqualified providers may pose a large financial burden, especially on poor and rural populations, with little or even negative health effects. Reducing or eliminating such practices is a daunting challenge. However, these same providers may offer opportunities for rapid expansion of coverage with certain essential services, if they can be properly trained, supervised, and supplied.

7.2.4.4 Conflicts of interest related to joint public/private sector practice. Multiple job-holding by physicians and paramedics is extremely common in many countries. Rent-seeking by private providers in public facilities, especially hospitals, has also been noted. Is the net social effect of these practices negative or positive? Should multiple job-holding be encouraged, although perhaps better regulated? To what extent do such arrangements result in substantial conflicts of interest on the parts of providers acting as agents for patients? To what extent do they lead to private appropriation of illicit profits from subsidies to public facilities?

7.3   SUPPLY-SIDE INTERVENTIONS TO IMPROVE PRIVATE HEALTH CARE

As noted above, there are sound theoretical reasons for expecting socially undesirable results from the unregulated development and operation of private health care. Experiences in many countries in Asia bear out these concerns, at least as far as anecdotal observation will take us. While more careful assessment of the performance of health care markets is needed to understand better the nature, size, and determinants of these effects, governments are already looking for remedies for current and future problems. What are the options available for public action and what can we learn from experiences to date?

Health sector development can be viewed as the result of the operation of a set of linked markets, as shown in Figure 7.1. A system such as that in Figure 7.1 is driven by the demand for health care services, such as hospital bed days and medical procedures. Such demand calls forth a supply of providers (doctors, hospitals, pharmacies). The actions of many individuals and institutions to create this supply creates in turn a demand for the inputs needed ("factors" in economic jargon), such as trained personnel, hospital buildings, and medical equipment. This process stimulates a market for inputs. Even the training of future medical personnel can be seen in this light, reflecting both the need for personnel from the supply side and the attractiveness of medical careers through expectations of future earnings, prestige, and security affecting the demand for, for example, medical education.

Of course, these markets are in reality far from the idealized economic model of perfect competition driven by the satisfaction of the needs of many individual consumers. It has already been noted that the initial level of demand for health care services may be significantly determined by the providers rather than the patients. Such provider-induced demand could result in production of more outputs than consumers would demand on their own. The existence of institutional payers also affects the operations of these markets and can result in excess supply (through unrestricted third-party payment) or constricted demand (through, for example, high levels of co-insurance or managed care). Institutions on the supply side also intervene in the market. For example, development of regulations for doctors and hospitals is often delegated by government to professional organizations (such as medical associations). These organizations may seek to advance the interests of their members through this mechanism. Economists have developed models of imperfect (monopolistic or oligopolistic) competition and other approaches to address these real world concerns.

Governments can take actions that affect the private health sector on both the demand and the supply side. Such actions can have short-run effects on private

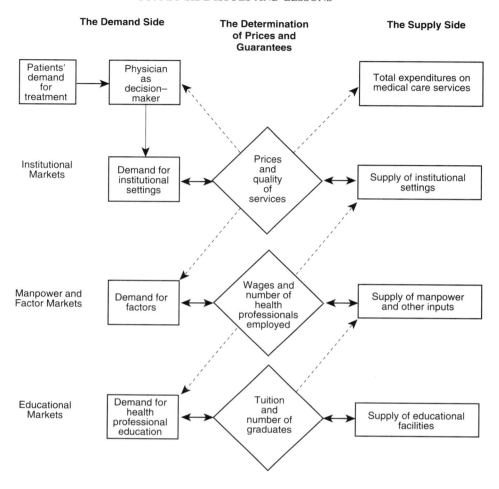

Figure 7.1. Linked Markets in the Health Sector. Reproduced from Feldstein (1993) by permission of Delmar Publications.

health care providers, altering the prices they charge and the quality and quantity of the services they provide. Interventions can also alter conditions over the longer run, in addition affecting the numbers and types of private providers, their location, and the types of facilities they create or operate.

Figure 7.2 presents graphically such effects of government action. Broadly, there are five types of government intervention that can affect the private health sector:

1. Government provision of health services directly
2. Government's direct financing of private providers
3. Indirect government fiscal actions that affect private provider's financing, such as taxes, duties on equipment, and subsidies for certain types of investment

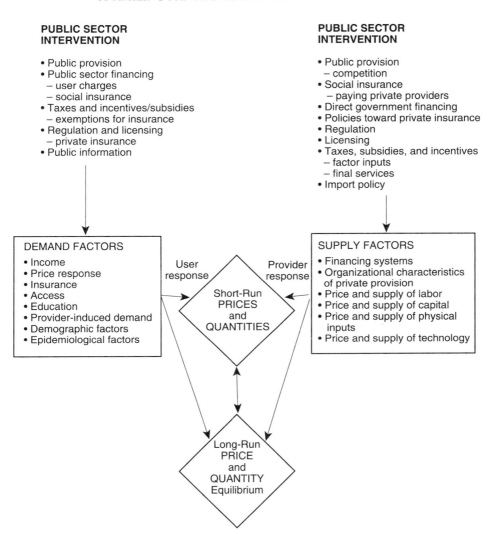

Figure 7.2. How Government Actions Affect Private Health Care. Note: Indirect public sector interventions, which are also important, are not represented in this figure. They include such interventions as provision of primary schooling, construction of roads and communications, and development of capital markets. These act predominantly via the demand side. Source: Berman and Rannan-Eliya (1993).

4. Legal and administrative actions of government, such as licensing of providers, legislation of legal liability, regulation of insurers, and quality regulation of private practice
5. Government provision of information to providers, users, and payers.

Not all of these will affect the supply side of the market, the focus of this chapter. The most important government interventions affecting the supply side are (2), (3), and (4) above, those that affect the financing of private health care, the costs of production, and the legal and regulatory environment. From these areas of intervention, three will be discussed: payment methods for private providers when they receive direct government or social insurance financing; indirect financing methods that provide incentives for production or affect the costs of inputs; and legal and regulatory actions.

7.4. PAYMENT METHODS AND PRIVATE PROVIDERS' BEHAVIOR

Health economists have devoted a great deal of effort to understanding the benefits and drawbacks of different approaches to paying health care providers. This has been one of the main approaches in health sector reform efforts that seek to contain costs (that is, increase efficiency), improve quality, and assure patient satisfaction.

For Asian countries, provider payment is likely to be a powerful tool for regulating private provider behavior. Typically, this has been a major concern in countries with social insurance schemes that pay private providers or are considering doing so. Opening up new sources of financing to the private health care sector offers the potential for expanding supply and access, but also contains the risks of costs and quality running out of control.

Another, as yet relatively untested, area for provider payment is for governments to pay private providers directly for services that governments want to make available. Private providers could substitute for government-owned providers in the delivery of a wide range of personal and public health services. As noted earlier, the large numbers of private providers in many Asian countries offer an opportunity for expanding coverage and access with priority services directly. Could provider payment methods be used to finance these new sources of care, while controlling the potentially undesirable effects?

In considering provider payment options, we should be thinking not only about the type of payment used but also about *who pays, what is paid for and at what price*, and *how provider output and quality are regulated* by the payer.

Figure 7.3 presents a commonly used representation of a tripartite health financing structure. In this simple model, the provider can be paid by the patient, or a third-party payer (such as a public or private insurance organization), or an employer. Financing—the payment for health care—is separated from the provision of the service. The provider can be and often is paid by more than one entity. Recent innovations have made one type of provider act as the payer for other providers. In the UK, for example, some general practitioners now manage budgets to pay hospitals for treatment of their patients referred for hospitalization. In other words, within this general framework, there are many alternatives, including some that blur the distinction between payer and provider, as do some new forms of health maintenance organizations in the USA.

In a recent review, Barnum *et al.* (1995) described four major methods of paying providers: fee-for-service, capitation, payment per case or per episode, and budgetary transfer. To these we might add salary-based payments to individual providers, which often coincide with budgetary transfers. (See the glossary for

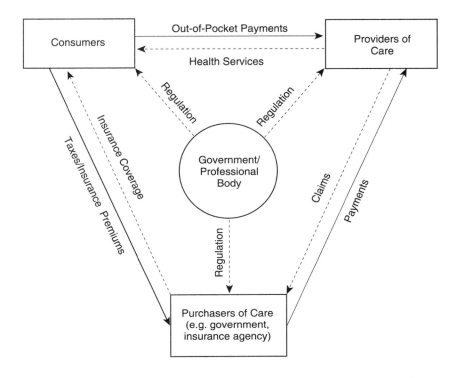

Figure 7.3. Tripartite Financing Arrangements for Health Care. Reproduced from World Health Organization (1994) with permission.

definitions of these different methods.) Each of these approaches to determining *what is paid for* results in different incentives to providers related to the quantity of cases they want to treat, the intensity of treatment in terms of the number of services or procedures given per case, the costs of production, and provider behavior in favoring certain types of patients over others. Table 7.2 summarizes the direction and strength of these effects for each individual payment method.

As is well known, no single payment method provides all the right incentives and different conditions. For example, in the USA, fee-for-service has been shown to encourage providers to increase the number of individual procedures billed for, with significant cost increases resulting from more quantity and intensity of care (Gabel and Redisch, 1979). However, in countries where provider productivity is very low, this might be an effective means of rapidly increasing output. Alternatively, capitation, while it does not encourage unnecessary procedures, gives providers an incentive to do less for patients, other things being equal. Their payment is not related to the quantity or quality of service provided, except to the extent that patients become so dissatisfied they seek another provider.

Intervening with changes in what is paid for may include changing not only the type of payment, but also the mix of services that are paid for with different methods.

Table 7.2. Summary of Incentives in Payment Methods.

	Underlying incentives for:			
Reimbursement type	Cost/unit	Services/case	Quantity (of cases)	Risk selection
Global budget	↓↓	↓↓	↓	0
FFS unconstrained	↓	↑↑	↑	0
FFS fixed	↓↓	↑↑	↑	↑
Capitation	↓↓	↓↓	↓↓	↑↑
Case based	↓↓	↓↓	↑↑	↑

↓↓, Strong incentive to reduce; ↓, moderate incentive to reduce; 0, no clear incentive; ↑, moderate incentive to increase; ↑↑, strong incentive to increase; FFS, fee-for-service.
Source: Barnum *et al.* (1995), Table 1.

For example, methods that provide strong incentives for increased output may be used for some highly desirable services (such as immunization), while other services are paid for in a different way.

Because no single payment method may be optimal, some economists have recommended using combinations of these approaches (Ma, 1994). In practice, in many systems providers already face a mixture of payment methods, but these may not be planned or regulated. For example, in many public facilities providers are paid by salary but may receive unofficial fee-for-service payments from patients. In some clinics and hospitals, official user fees may be utilized in part as supplementary bonus payments to staff; these payments may or may not be tied to output.

Who pays may also be important, since payers face different incentives that affect their choice of payment method and their ability and willingness to pursue the benefits of different approaches. For example, in the USA, third-party payers (mainly private insurers) face strong incentives to control costs in order to maintain profits in a highly competitive environment. Their pursuit of savings, however, is modulated by the need to keep providers and patients satisfied. In contrast, in the UK, some general practitioners have now been delegated responsibility as payers for hospital care under the recent National Health Service reforms. They also face incentives to control costs, but their close personal links to individual patients may have different results than if payments were being made by an institutional third party.

In order to derive the benefits from payment methods, and to reduce any negative effects, any payer should be concerned about the management and regulation of their provider payments. Setting payment rates or prices, making sure payments are made promptly and appropriately, and monitoring the quantity and quality of services provided all require extensive data, analysis, and systematic decision-making. All approaches are also vulnerable to fraud and abuse. Their demands on institutional capacity may differ for different payment methods. For example, payment per service or per case may require more extensive record-keeping, reporting, and monitoring than, for example, salary or capitation-based payments. Barnum *et al.* (1995) point out that the information and administrative requirements for the proper use of some payment methods may be well beyond the capacities of countries without well-developed health care administrations.

7.4.1 Recent experiences

7.4.1.1 Korea: mixed payments system under partial national health insurance. The Republic of Korea instituted national health insurance in 1977 and has gradually expanded coverage to reach 94 per cent of the population by 1992. Over the same period, private health care provision has also increased, with private and non-profit facilities accounting for 95 per cent of hospitals and 91 per cent of beds in 1994. (See Chapter 5 and Yang, 1990, 1991, 1995.)

Yang describes the mixed payment system facing most providers and patients. National health insurance pays providers on a fee-for-service basis, with significant deductibles and co-insurance paid by the patients (see Chapter 4). Provider fees for covered services, most of the outpatient services and inpatient services, are regulated and set on a cost-plus basis at a level that allows most providers to earn profits. However, providers are also permitted to charge patients for uncovered services, for which the fees are not regulated and for which, it is assumed, profits could be much larger. Uncovered services include new and expensive high technology such as CT scans and ultrasonography. Patients may also be asked to pay special treatment charges to be treated by a specialist in hospital. Many providers also sell drugs as part of their practice. These additional services are not covered by insurance.

According to Yang, the incentive faced by providers to increase the quantity of uncovered services has had several effects. First, total health spending has increased rapidly. Yet despite the expansion of national health insurance coverage, household out-of-pocket payments still account for over 60 per cent of total health expenditure. Second, providers have rapidly increased their investments in new medical technologies, especially those not covered by insurance payments. Charges for these services are high, at 300 to 600 per cent of estimated costs for the services studied. Third, drug consumption, stimulated by private provider incentives and largely unregulated, has kept pace with increased spending and accounts for about 30 per cent of total health expenditure. Fourth, the financial burden of uncovered services may be greater for lower-income families than for better-off families.

7.4.1.2 The Philippines: problems in regulating provider payment under health insurance. Formal health insurance in the Philippines is provided under the Medicare program, which in 1991 covered about 39 per cent of the population. Medicare provides only inpatient benefits, covering both hospital and physician services associated with an inpatient episode. Full coverage is provided up to a ceiling, above which patients pay out-of-pocket. Medicare has maximum per-item allowances for payments for specific hospital services and for specific physician services. Solon *et al.* (1995) describe how the room charge allowance, for example, is always less than the prevailing room charges. However, providers face incentives to increase the quantity of specific services, as well as the charges for those services. Charges, up to the maximum allowed, are essentially free-of-charge to the patient.

Beyond the allowance, the patient may still be willing to pay up to a point where the marginal benefit to the patient would exceed the out-of-pocket cost.

Using 1993 data, the study compared the charges for hospital and physician services from a sample of public and private sector facilities. The comparison included detailed information on the type of facility, quantity and types of services received, total charges, and personal and socioeconomic characteristics of the patients. One objective was to determine whether a patient's eligibility for insurance gave a signal to providers that they could charge more for a given service, since insurance payments were available. Such price discrimination on the part of providers, if possible, would certainly increase the attractiveness of insured patients to providers. However, the increased payments for insured patients would also in effect be a transfer of resources from the patients (via the payer) to the providers for no additional real benefit. It would result in higher premiums to patients and higher incomes to providers, with higher health expenditures than would be the case without this behavior.

For hospital charges, the study reported no price effect of insurance coverage from publicly owned facilities, but a significant effect in privately owned hospitals, equivalent on average to a 20 per cent mark-up for insured patients. Physician's services were found to have a 50 per cent mark-up for insured patients. Overall, such mark-ups would account for a significant percentage of total Medicare benefits.

The Medicare payment method, maximum per-service allowances, is vulnerable to such discriminatory behavior unless the payer is able to monitor differences in charges for insured and uninsured patients. Private providers had both the incentive and capability to respond to this opportunity. The study suggests that this results in increased costs and welfare losses to the insured population. However, price discrimination may have social benefits and it is also possible that such behavior results in a greater quantity of services provided overall and at lower prices to the uninsured. The study did not analyze the possible provider response in unnecessarily increasing the quantity of services to the insured population.

7.5   INDIRECT FINANCING INTERVENTIONS

Indirect financing interventions include two categories of public sector action: (1) financial interventions that affect the cost and availability of various inputs (medical personnel, drugs, and equipment) in the provision of health care services; and (2) financial interventions that encourage or discourage the provision of certain health care services. These interventions are indirect since they operate through the provider's decision-making process. They contrast with the action of government or other payers simply to pay directly for private service provision, as discussed above.

Creating medical care capacity requires costly investments, including lengthy and expensive training of physicians and nurses, buildings for hospitals and clinics, and, increasingly, high-cost equipment. In addition, the provision of health services requires reliable access to supplies such as drugs. These inputs may need to be imported, requiring foreign exchange and making them relatively costly in local

Table 7.3. Examples of Input Subsidies to Private Providers.

Type of input	Example of subsidy
Trained medical, nursing, and auxiliary personnel	Free or low-cost education in publicly financed institutions, with little or no requirement of public service thereafter
Medical equipment and supplies	Manufacture and sale below cost from government-owned production facilities
	Low import duties
	Foreign exchange subsidies for imports
Ambulatory care practice	By allowing private practice for government providers, the risk of developing new practice is reduced and some initial costs are subsidized (space, equipment, vehicle, etc.)
Hospitals	Allowing private providers to admit private patients to public hospitals, charging market rates for physician services but subsidized prices for hospital services
Capital	Publicly guaranteed and subsidized lending for private investment in hospitals, clinics
	Tax incentives for private individual and corporate investment in, or donations to, medical facilities

terms. Table 7.3 gives some examples of different kinds of input subsidies commonly found in developing countries.

In many developing countries, the government has led the way in making the large investments needed to create health care capacity and in creating conditions that reduce barriers to access to recurrent inputs. Medical schools and hospitals are often predominantly owned by governments. Governments have developed drug and equipment manufacturing capacity and intervene in the import and marketing of these inputs.

Such interventions were initially justified as part of social policies to assure access to health care for all. However, governments have often been unwilling or unable to capture all the benefits from these public investments for public purposes. For some types of investments, such as medical education, this is difficult to do without very restrictive personnel policies (such as requiring long periods of public service). As a result, private health care providers benefit from a wide variety of public subsidies to inputs. In addition, some governments are now formally promoting private health care development.

It is likely that these subsidies significantly affect the pattern and pace of private health care development. For example, private medical practice has tended to develop first in ambulatory care, where investments are much more modest, there are subsidies from joint public/private practice, and public hospitals provide subsidized referral capacity. Private investment in smaller and then larger hospitals can follow (Berman and Rannan-Eliya, 1993).

Governments have paid little attention to date to the size of these subsidies overall and the relative gains to public and private actors. Governments could also try to make better use of these subsidies to further public sector health objectives.

Another area of public action concerns incentives to private providers to encourage them to increase the output of specific types of services. This approach has been used extensively in national family planning programs, where private physicians may receive training and free or subsidized supplies and equipment. Other examples include provision of free vaccines, and training and supplies for treating specific diseases such as diarrhea, STDs, respiratory infections, and tuberculosis.

7.5.1 Recent experiences

7.5.1.1 Thailand: government support for private hospital investment. Mongkolsmai (Chapter 6) and Nittayaramphong and Tangcharoensathien (1994) document the rapid growth of private hospitals in Thailand beginning in the mid-1970s. This trend coincided with and was encouraged by a broader national strategy of encouraging private sector growth. Private hospitals and beds have increased as a percentage of the national total since the 1970s. This is associated with an increase in household out-of-pocket expenditure in total national health spending, increased private practice by physicians, and rising quantities of high-technology medical equipment.

An important factor in this growth, it is argued, was support from the Board of Investment (BOI) through its Hotels and Hospitals Division and from the Ministry of Finance. These agencies helped by providing corporate tax holidays, waivers for import taxes, and financial support for construction of new private hospitals. Expanded support from the BOI is closely associated with increases in hospital supply in Bangkok. Although it was not possible to attribute a specific share of the growth in private hospitals to this type of support, the authors called for better integration of such investment assistance with national health policy goals.

7.5.1.2 Indonesia: partially subsidized contraceptives for the middle classes. Indonesia has been seeking to reduce its budgetary burden for the procurement of expendable supplies in family planning (Kenney, 1989). Noting significant and increasing use of private providers to obtain contraceptives by urban and middle-class women, the national family program has tried marketing partially subsidized contraceptives, which would be used primarily by private providers with their paying patients. These "Blue Circle" supplies would substitute for the completely subsidized family planning supplies available from public clinics and facilities.

While these supplies have been picked up by many private providers, it has proven difficult to reduce the leakage of free supplies from the public program to the private providers, since many providers work in both sectors. Uptake has been gradual. Despite the desire of many middle-class women for services outside the public system, private family planning services are fairly costly in comparison to highly subsidized government services.

7.6 LEGAL AND REGULATORY INTERVENTIONS AFFECTING PRIVATE PROVIDERS

Legal and regulatory interventions can affect the costs and availability of inputs needed by private providers, the prices of the services they produce, the quantity and distribution of private services, and the quality of services (see Chapter 10). Laws may be used to set broader directions and intent and to empower agents of the state to regulate, while regulations and the regulatory actions of different agencies generally encompass the more detailed applications of laws in specific settings. These legal interventions are typically coercive and used to restrict undesirable behavior, in contrast to indirect financing interventions, whose intent is persuasive, rather than coercive, and which are used to encourage desirable behavior.

Effective regulation requires sufficient state capacity to collect information, devise sound rules, and monitor and enforce compliance. Capacities in these areas have typically been weak in developing countries. Underpaid civil servants may lack zeal in enforcing regulations. Courts of law may also not be very effective in providing rapid and consistent remedies. There are ample opportunities for corruption and co-optation of the regulators by the regulated.

Because of the technical and professional nature of medical practice, there has typically been close involvement of the medical profession in developing laws and regulations and in their application. For example, national or regional (state or province level) medical associations — private bodies — are usually given formal state recognition and may be empowered to establish licensing and registration procedures for physicians and hospitals. They may also be charged with investigating professional malfeasance and applying sanctions. This self-policing role of professional bodies has often been criticized as regulatory capture.

Direct price regulation is typically not used for health care services by private physicians or hospitals. However, governments may attempt to regulate private sector prices through price-setting for comparable public sector services. Where there is effective competition between public and private providers, this can serve to limit private provider behavior. This approach has allegedly been effective in Malaysia. In the People's Republic of China, the government continues to regulate the prices of some services provided by largely autonomous hospitals and clinics. This has been noted to encourage use of nonregulated services (Liu et al., 1994). A similar effect was noted earlier through the partial price-setting of national health insurance in Korea.

Price regulation has been used extensively for pharmaceuticals. In India, for example, the government has identified several broad classes of pharmaceuticals and applied different degrees of price control to each class. Those drugs classed as most essential for treating common diseases are subject to strict controls of wholesale and retail prices. Maximum retail prices are clearly marked on product containers. Manufacturers and providers have argued that this practice may encourage production and prescription of less controlled items.

Regulation is more apparent in efforts to affect the quantity and quality of private providers (see Chapter 10). Governments generally endeavor to license individual providers, both physicians and other allied health workers such as midwives, nurses, and pharmacists, as well as health care facilities, including hospitals, pharmacies, laboratories, and diagnostic-testing facilities. Licensing may include setting standards for buildings, equipment, and staffing. Regulation of the actions of these providers includes, for example, restricting the dispensing of certain pharmaceuticals without a physician's prescription.

In many Asian countries, these efforts at regulation are largely ineffective, due to totally inadequate capacity for enforcement. In India, unqualified medical practitioners (not including traditional practitioners) in open private practice vastly outnumber those with proper qualifications, perhaps by as much as three to one (Vishwanathan, 1994). State governments, which are legally responsible for licensing and registration, lack up-to-date figures on both qualified and unqualified practitioners. A recent study in one Indian state identified almost twice as many private hospital beds as were officially registered with government authorities. Registration systems are terribly out-of-date, both in terms of registering new practitioners as well as removing from local lists those who are deceased or who have relocated (see Chapter 8).

The inability of many governments to regulate retail pharmaceutical distribution is also well known. Drugs that should be available only with a physician's prescription are often easily obtainable over the counter. Drug manufacturing standards are difficult to enforce and spurious drugs are often widely available.

Another important element of government regulation in Asia concerns the rules affecting private use of public resources in the health sector. One dimension of this is related to multiple job-holding by government-employed providers. A second aspect is the rules affecting use of government-owned hospitals and related facilities by private practitioners.

Part-time private practice by government-employed physicians is widespread in Asia. In theory, this could have both positive and negative effects on patients and public sector programs (Ellis and Chawla, 1993). There has been little research to investigate the dynamics of such joint practice and to determine how government rules could reduce the undesirable outcomes.

The second problem, private appropriation of the benefits of the public subsidies in government-owned hospitals, has also been given little formal attention. Often, physicians with privileges in higher-level government hospitals also maintain a private practice. They may be able to admit their private patients in these facilities, earning private fees for themselves while obtaining significant subsidies for their patients for hospital and other services. Such arrangements may be an important factor attracting physicians to affiliate with public hospitals or even maintain part-time public employment. Should government regulate this practice?

Legal interventions can also include laws empowering consumers to take action against providers for malpractice, or laws restricting such actions. (The recent experience of India is cited below.) However, this area of public action has not been well documented to date.

7.6.1 Recent experiences

7.6.1.1 The Consumer Protection Act in India.   India recently permitted application of its Consumer Protection Act to the provision of private medical services. Under the provisions of this Act, individual complainants can bring legal action against private practitioners in special consumer courts. These courts are much more accessible to the public than the regular courts. Cases are heard relatively quickly after filing and rulings are expected more rapidly.

Bhat (see Chapter 8 and Bhat, 1993a) found a high level of awareness about these regulations among private practitioners. Providers were concerned that they would now be more vulnerable to legal action and that this would result in increased health care costs to consumers.

7.7 CONCLUSION

There is a widespread perception in Asia that private sector health care provision is growing rapidly. Some perceive this to pose significant problems for national health care systems. It is feared that expanding private health care will cause rapid cost escalation, reduced equity, and poor-quality or inappropriate health care. It also may threaten the capacity for public sector services to expand as needed. Government action is needed immediately to address these problems and to channel private sector growth in directions that will reduce its negative effects and enhance its capacity to support national health goals.

Others perceive new opportunities in the expansion of private health care provision capacity. These opportunities are not just about reallocating government resources away from higher-level urban care to primary health care priorities. They also include the potential to use the substantial existing capacity of private providers to expand coverage and access to essential basic services of good quality at a cost equal to or below current government provision costs.

Is private sector growth the problem many have claimed? The experiences of other countries suggest that it certainly could be, although we probably do not have sufficient information to generalize at this time. However, Asian countries can learn from both the positive and negative experiences of the wealthier countries. These suggest that market failures in the health sector can result in highly undesirable outcomes for health care efficiency and equity; there are, nonetheless, important social benefits from the operation of market-like forces in health care; and appropriate public action in the areas of financing, provision, regulation, and information can be successful in creating conditions where the ownership of health care facilities *per se* is not very important.

Government–private sector collaboration has only just begun to explore the opportunities offered. Family planning and a few public health programs have tried to expand their coverage through involvement of private providers, but often using only those in the formal sector and in cities. These efforts could be much more ambitious geographically and programmatically. A few governments have also been systematically shifting the burden of higher-level services to private providers. There is concern about the ability to control costs and assure quality in many of these efforts.

This chapter has focused on the potential interventions that affect private health care provision from the supply side. A complete view requires harmonization of both supply- and demand-side policies. Even this partial view suggests that there is much that can be done to influence private health care provision in ways that control costs, encourage appropriate levels of quantity and quality of services, and increase consumer satisfaction.

At this time, most countries in Asia lack sufficient information to define clearly the problems and issues they face regarding the development of private sector health care. A better description of the situation and a sound diagnosis of the relevant conditions should be a high priority for those concerned about this issue.

Even with inadequate information and analysis, many countries already face a complex environment of public action affecting the financing and regulation of private health care. They need to move ahead simultaneously to refine policies and actions affecting the private health sector and to monitor and evaluate their impact.

Countries should not need to address these issues entirely on their own. There are important lessons that countries in the region can learn from each other, as they develop and expand new forms of public and private health care financing and address the challenges of rapid changes in demand and technology. And there may be gains from collaboration in the region to improve laws, regulations, and information systems. Regional organizations such as the Asian Development Bank can assist in this process, as can other groupings of countries in the region such as the Association of South East Asian Nations and the South Asia Association for Regional Cooperation.

Most countries in Asia have accepted the principle of pluralism in health care provision, in fact if not always as planned. Private health sector growth undoubtedly involves both problems and opportunities. The challenge is how to reap the most social benefits in the future from the realities of today, increasing the positive and reducing the negative. In health care, this will clearly require government action. An impressive array of tools and methods are available, needing only adequate knowledge and the will to apply them.

REFERENCES

Barnum, H., Kutzin, J., Saxenian, H. (1995). *Incentives and Provider Payment Methods.* HRO Working Paper No. 5. Washington, DC: World Bank.

Bennett, S. (1992). Promoting the private sector: a review of developing country trends. *Health Policy and Planning,* 7(2), 97–110.

Berman, P., Rannan-Eliya, R. (1993). *Factors Affecting the Development of Private Health Care Provision in Developing Countries.* Major Applied Research Paper No. 9. Bethesda, MD: Health Financing and Sustainability Project.

Bhat, R. (1993a). The private health care sector in India. In: Berman, P., Kahn, M. (Eds). *Paying for India's Health Care.* New Delhi: Sage Publications.

Bhat, R. (1993b). The private/public mix in health care in India. *Health Policy and Planning,* 8(1), 43–56.

Ellis, R., Chawla, M. (1993). *Public and Private Interactions in the Health Sector in Developing Countries.* Major Applied Research Paper No. 5. Bethesda, MD: Health Financing and Sustainability Project.

Feldstein, P.J. (1993). *Health Care Economics.* Albany, NY: Delmar Publications.

Gabel, J., Redisch, M. (1979). Alternative physician payment methods: incentives, efficiency, and national health insurance. *Milbank Memorial Fund Quarterly,* **57**, 1.

Griffin, C., Alano, B., Ginson-Bautista, M., Gamboa, R. (1994). *The Private Medical Sector in the Philippines.* HFDP Monograph No. 4. Manila, Philippines: Department of Health.

Hsiao, W. (1995). Abnormal economics in the health sector. In: Berman, P. (Ed.). *Health Sector Reform in Developing Countries: Making Health Development Sustainable.*

Cambridge, MA: Harvard University Press, 161–182. Also published in *Health Policy*, **32**(1–3), 161–179.

Kenney, G. (1989). *The Economics of Private Sector Family Planning Service Provision in Indonesia*. Publication No. 3847-01. Washington, DC: Urban Institute.

Liu, G., Liu, X., Meng, X. (1994). Privatization of the medical market in socialist China: a historical approach. *Health Policy*, **27**, 157–174.

Ma, C. (1994). Health care payment systems: cost and quality incentives. *Journal of Economics and Management Strategy*, **3**, 1.

National Health Survey. (1993). Ministry of Health, People's Republic of China.

Nittayaramphong, S., Tangcharoensathien, V. (1994). Thailand: private health care out of control? *Health Policy and Planning*, **9**(1), 31–40.

Organization for Economic Cooperation and Development (OECD). (1995). *Internal Markets in the Making: Health Systems in Canada, Iceland and the United Kingdom*. Health Policy Studies No. 6. Paris: OECD.

Paqueo, V., Lieberman, S. (1992). *Indonesia: Health Insurance Issues in the 1990s*. Draft.

Rohde, E., Vishwanathan, H. 1995. *The Rural Private Practitioner*. New Delhi: Oxford University Press.

Patao, D., Jeffers, J. (1994). *Profile of Medicare Program II Target Beneficiaries*. Health Finance Development Project Monograph No. 8. Manila: Philippines Department of Health, USAID, and Management Sciences for Health.

Smutharaks, B. (1993). *Assessing Thailand's Health Care Financing System*. Background document for workshop on Health Financing, November 12–13, 1993, Thailand.

Solon, O., Gertler, P., Alabastro, S. (1995). *Insurance and Price Discrimination in the Market for Hospital Services in the Philippines*. Paper presented at the Asian Development Bank First Regional Conference on Health Sector Reform in Asia, May 22–25, 1995, Manila.

Thomason, J. (1992). *Collaborative Research Group on the Public/Private Mix: Papua New Guinea Country Paper*. Department of Community Medicine, University of Papua New Guinea.

Vishwanathan, H. (1994). *The Rural Private Practitioner*. New Delhi, India: Social and Rural Research Unit, and Market Research Bureau.

World Bank. (1995). *World Development Report 1995: Workers in an Integrating World*. New York: Oxford University Press.

World Health Organization (WHO). (1994). *Evaluation of Recent Changes in the Financing of Health Services*. WHO Technical Report Series No. 829. Geneva: WHO.

Yang, B. (1990). *Issues in Health Care Delivery: the Case of Korea*. Paper presented at a World Bank meeting on health insurance, December 1990, Bali, Indonesia.

Yang, B. (1991). Health insurance in Korea: opportunities and challenges. *Health Policy and Planning*, **6**(2), 119–129.

Yang, B. (1995). *Health Care System of Korea: What Now and What in the Future?* Paper presented at the Asian Development Bank First Regional Conference on Health Sector Reform in Asia, May 22–25, 1995, Manila.

8

Regulation of The Private Health Sector in India

RAMESH BHAT

Professor, Indian Institute of Management

8.1 INTRODUCTION

The private sector plays an important role in India's health care delivery system. Through a wide network of health care facilities, this sector caters to the needs of both urban and rural populations and has expanded widely to meet increasing demands. Utilization patterns indicate that health care seekers depend highly on the private sector (Duggal and Amin, 1989; Yesudian, 1990). Despite the widespread public facilities, a higher proportion of health services is provided by the private sector than by government facilities (Chatterjee, 1988).

The private health care sector has grown significantly. The growth of this sector has been triggered by a number of factors, including a new national economic policy, the rapid influx of medical technology, growing deficits of public sector hospitals, and a rising middle class. Its growth has profound implications for the character of the current Indian health care system and its future course.

Recent studies indicate that private health care significantly affects both the cost and quality of health care services in India (Uplekar, 1989a,b; Duggal and Amin, 1989; Vishwanathan and Rohde, 1990; Yesudian, 1990). Although cases of superfluous and excessively high-cost services rendered by private physicians and hospitals have been reported (Uplekar, 1989a,b; Duggal and Amin, 1989), there is no evidence that these result in any greater use of public facilities.

Significantly, despite the problems resulting from the rapid growth of the private sector, there has been little effort to establish market or regulatory mechanisms to ensure its appropriate growth. This is unfortunate, since it is well known that leaving health care to market forces does not necessarily lead to an effective and efficient health care system (see Chapter 2).

The role of the state and self-regulating bodies is important in minimizing the unintended and undesirable consequences emanating from the growth of the private sector. At some point, it becomes imperative for the stakeholders to address the

Private Health Sector Growth in Asia: Issues and Implications. Edited by W. Newbrander.

issues of equity, efficiency, and quality of care in this sector. This chapter considers the role of these stakeholders in addressing such concerns. It specifically discusses: the status of existing regulation (self-regulation or government legislation) to monitor and control private health sector practices; the performance of these laws in ensuring the appropriate development of this sector; and the issues and problems experienced in implementing regulations, through case studies of three important regulations.

After describing the broad characteristics of the private health sector in India, this chapter examines the major policy concerns originating from its growth. It assesses the current regulatory environment and its implications for the process of health reform.

The description of the private health sector includes information about the share of the private sector in the total health care infrastructure, the characteristics of the private sector in terms of the scale and scope of operations, utilization patterns of private services, aggregate and per capita expenditure on private health care, and the methods of financing used by households for these expenditures.

The assessment of the current regulatory environment includes three case studies: on the Consumer Protection Act (COPRA); the Medical Council of India (MCI) and state medical councils (SMCs) in India; and, on the Nursing Home Act (NHA).

8.2   PRIVATE HEALTH CARE SERVICES

The structure of the health care system in India is complex and includes various types of providers. These providers practise in different systems of medicines and facilities. The providers and facilities in India can be broadly classified by using three dimensions: ownership styles (public, private not-for-profit, private for-profit and private informal); systems of medicine (allopathic, homeopathic, and traditional); and types of facilities (hospitals, dispensaries, and clinics). These dimensions are interdependent and overlapping (Bhat, 1993).

Using the ownership criterion, the health care system can be divided into four broad sectors: (1) the public sector, including government-run hospitals, dispensaries, clinics, primary health care centers and subcenters, and paramedics; (2) the private not-for-profit sector, including voluntary health programs, charitable institutions, missions, churches, and trusts; (3) the organized private for-profit sector, including general practitioners (having at least a bachelor's degree or equivalent in medicine), private hospitals and dispensaries (popularly known as nursing homes), registered medical practitioners, and other licensed practitioners; and (4) the private informal sector, including practitioners without formal qualifications (such as faith healers, herbalists, priests, *tantriks*, *hakims*, and *vaidyas*).

8.2.1   *Government policy on private health care services*

Improving public health for all is recorded as one of the primary duties of the state in the Indian constitution. To achieve this goal, the planning process of the country allows the states to develop their health services infrastructure, as well as facilities for medical education and research.

Since the inception of the planning process, the state and central governments have experienced a number of constraints in implementing health programs effectively. In 1982, the National Health Policy (NHP) acknowledged these constraints and suggested an integrated and comprehensive approach for the future development of health care services.

To mitigate the problem of limited resources, the policy document recommended that the states should design processes to encourage practice by private medical professionals and investment by nongovernmental agencies in establishing curative centers. States were also encouraged to provide organizational, logistical, financial, and technical support to voluntary agencies active in the health field.

The NHP's emphasis on promoting private and voluntary health curative services has been an important step toward providing clear direction to the states. Planning to help state governments develop their own strategies to utilize untapped resources and strengthen their ability to meet the growing health needs of their people has been carried out through the NHP process.

8.2.2 Facilities

According to information available about the distribution of hospitals and hospital beds according to ownership (see Table 8.1), about 57 per cent of the 11 174 hospitals are in the private sector. In 1992, the private sector owned about 32 per cent of the total hospital bed capacity, while the government and local government agencies owned the other 68 per cent. About 60 per cent of total reported dispensaries are in the private sector, with about 32 per cent of the bed capacity.

The data on hospital bed capacity show that the majority of private hospitals are smaller than public ones (Bhat, 1993). About 85 per cent of the hospitals in the private sector have a capacity of fewer than 25 beds. These facilities account for about 40 per cent of the hospital bed capacity in the private sector. The average capacity of these hospitals is about 10 beds.

Analysis shows significant variation in expenditure (for example, per-bed total expenditure and per-bed salary expenditure) across the various size and ownership categories (Satia and Deodhar, 1993). Salary expenditures as a percentage of total expenditures also vary significantly.

As for the geographic distribution of health care facilities, Table 8.2 provides information on distribution by percentage of urban and rural hospitals and hospital beds belonging to the public and private sectors. The data show that about 69 per cent of the total hospitals are in urban areas. The distribution of hospital beds is similarly urban biased. The urban hospitals provide about 84 per cent of the total bed capacity. Private hospitals are relatively less urban biased: about 36 per cent of private hospitals and 29 per cent of their beds are in rural areas, compared to only 25 per cent of government hospitals and 10 per cent of their beds.

The growth of the private sector, as reflected in the number of hospitals and hospital bed capacity, is quite significant: during the last 10 years, the number of hospitals has doubled and bed capacity has grown by more than 50 per cent.

Table 8.1. Hospitals and Dispensaries by Ownership, 1992.

Ownership	Hospital and hospital beds				Dispensaries and dispensary beds			
	Hospitals	Per cent	Beds	Per cent	Dispensaries	Per cent	Beds	Per cent
Government								
Central and state	4411	40	411 868	64	8587	31	13 378	61
Local	346	3	23 347	4	2481	9	1617	7
Private	6417	57	206 888	32	16 363	60	7063	32
Total	11 174	100	642 103	100	27 431	100	22 058	100

Source: Directorate of Health Services and CMIE, Basic Statistics, August 1994.

Table 8.2. Distribution of Hospitals and Hospital Beds in Rural and Urban Areas by Ownership, 1988.

	Government		Private		Total	
	Number	Per cent	Number	Per cent	Number	Per cent
Hospitals						
Rural	1038	25	1928	36	2966	31
Urban	3176	75	3461	64	6637	69
Total	4214	100	5389	100	9603	100
Hospital beds						
Rural	39 154	10	49 930	29	89 084	16
Urban	363 026	90	121 468	71	484 494	84
Total	402 180	100	171 398	100	573 578	100

Source: Directory of Hospitals in India, 1988.

However, it should be noted that the number of hospitals, dispensaries, and doctors operating in the private sector is underreported. Many institutions in the private sector, including nursing homes and private clinics, are not covered by these health statistics.

8.2.3 Providers

According to a study by the Foundation for Research in Community Health (Jesani and Anantharam, 1989), about 242 650 qualified physicians in the allopathic system of medicine were practising privately, as compared to 88 105 in government services. Using information available for only a few states, one finds significant variation across regions in the number of physicians practising privately. Table 8.3 shows the number of doctors registered with the medical councils in India and the number of doctors working in government health care institutions in some of the states and union territories.

The total number of doctors registered with medical councils was 389 898 in 1991 in the 16 states for which data are available. The number of doctors employed with government agencies at the end of 1991 totalled 78 373 registered doctors. From these data, we find that about 80 per cent of the registered doctors are working in the private sector.

There are also large numbers of health care providers practising in other systems of medicines. Data from the state of Gujarat (1987 to 1993) found that about 50 per cent of the providers belong to systems of medicine other than allopathic, such as

Table 8.3. Physician Providers by State, 1991.

State	Population served per government doctor	Doctors registered with medical councils	Number of government doctors
Andhra Pradesh	61 471	32 931	1059
Arunachal Pradesh	3536	NA	233
Assam	8750	10 497	2660
Bihar	15 438	26 374	5238
Gao	2166	NA	540
Gujarat	11 404	21 812	3645
Haryana	11 705	523	1401
Himichal Pradesh	5350	NA	952
Jammu & Kashmir	5350	4307	1331
Karnataka	13 536	44 183	3397
Kerala	7213	16 455	4163
Madhya Pradesh	6418	11 187	9791
Maharashtra	11 404	49 365	6497
Manipur	2675	NA	684
Meghalaya	5357	NA	322
Mizoram	5000	NA	146
Nagaland	5401	NA	202
Orissa	6418	11 089	4965
Punjab	5642	26 636	3462
Rajasthan	NA	14 046	2156
Sikkim	4297	NA	101
Tamil Nadu	17 879	45 588	3189
Tripura	3822	NA	673
Uttar Pradesh	15 438	33 178	8630
West Bengal	6418	41 727	10 068
Union Territories			
Andaman	3448	NA	122
Chandigarh	913	NA	864
Dadra & Nagar	11 000	NA	12
Daman & Diu	5346	NA	19
Delhi	6233	NA	1473
Lakshadweep	1714	NA	28
Pondicherry	2174	NA	350
Total		389 898	78 373

NA, Not applicable.
Sources: Centre for Monitoring Indian Economy; and Health Information of India, Central Bureaus of Health Intelligence, Directorate of Health and Family Welfare, Government of India.

homeopathic, ayurvedic and unani. Most of them are private practitioners in rural areas.

In addition, there is a large number of unqualified providers who are engaged in providing health care services. Vishwanathan and Rohde (1990) found that about 62 per cent of the private doctors identified in the survey had no formal medical qualifications.

8.3   UTILIZATION OF PRIVATE HEALTH CARE SERVICES

Studies on utilization patterns show that people generally prefer private health care facilities. In a study by Duggal and Amin (1989) of 590 households in the Jalgaon district of Maharashtra, patients chose not-for-profit and for-profit private practitioners and hospitals for 77 per cent of their illness episodes and government-run facilities for only 13 per cent. National surveys indicate that private providers are the main providers of ambulatory health care, accounting for about 75 per cent of utilization. Vishwanathan and Rohde (1990) found that 65 per cent of diarrhea patients chose private medical consultations.

The evidence suggests that differences in income or location (rural versus urban) do not influence the use of different types of facilities. Private health care services are utilized by all social classes. Yesudian (1990), in a survey of the utilization of health facilities by people living in two slum communities in Bombay, found that people in both communities used private sector facilities more frequently for short-term and minor ailments. However, in acute cases of illnesses requiring hospitalization, they used public facilities, primarily for cost rather than quality considerations.

8.4   THE COST OF PRIVATE HEALTH CARE

8.4.1   Expenditures

Surveys on household expenditures indicate that spending on health care as a proportion of total consumption is significant: it is estimated at 7 to 9 per cent. The data also show that government expenditures in the health sector are small in proportion to what is being spent by households.

Public expenditure on health care in India is composed of spending by central government, state governments, and local bodies. Private health care spending includes the out-of-pocket costs incurred by households and expenditure by the private nonhousehold institutional sector. Their share of total health expenditure in 1984–85 was 63 per cent (Satia et al., 1987). Central, state, and local government account for the remaining 37 per cent of health expenditure. In a 1970 study, household and other private expenditures were estimated to be as high as 84 per cent of total health expenditure (de Ferranti, 1985).

Total health expenditure as a percentage of gross domestic product (GDP) was about 5 per cent. Due to increased demand for health care services over the years, this percentage of GDP has risen.

Expenditures on health amounted to Rs. 2050 million in 1960–61 and increased to Rs. 98 370 million in 1992–93. As shown in Figure 8.1, per capita private expenditure on health has increased at a rate of 12.5 per cent per year.

As the GDP has increased, per capita private health care expenditure has increased at a faster rate, as shown in Figure 8.2. The income elasticity is 1.47, which means that for each 1 per cent increase in per capita income, the private expenditure on health increased by 1.47 per cent. Much of this growth in the private sector in India can be attributed to the growth in incomes over the period.

8.4.2 Financing

Financing of health care by sources outside the household, such as insurance, has been minimal. Only 4 per cent of total health expenditure (Rs. 7.50 per capita per year) was found to be reimbursed by employers in Jalgaon (Duggal and Amin, 1989). The study also observed that people borrowed about Rs. 29 per capita per year (about 16 per cent of total health care expenditure) to finance their health costs. In some cases, borrowing was as high as their annual incomes.

Insurance coverage for health care expenses is very limited in India. Although the government initiated comprehensive health insurance schemes for employees in the government and formal private sectors, these schemes cover only 4 per cent of workers.

Recently, the national insurance companies have started selling individual medical insurance policies, but without much success. By 1989, 3 years after its launch, the

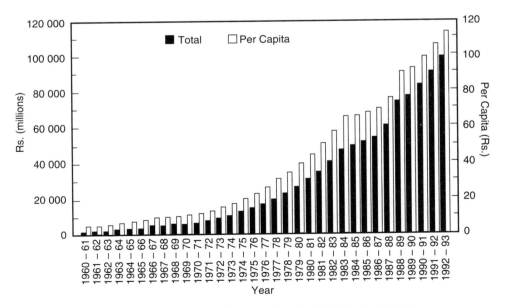

Figure 8.1. Private Expenditure on Health, 1960–61 to 1992–93.

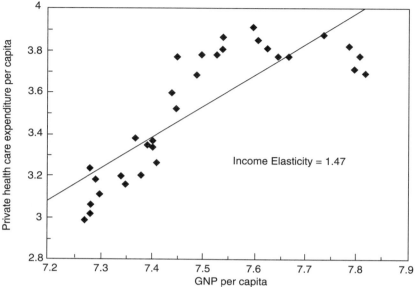

Figure 8.2. Private Health Care Expenditure and Gross National Product per Capita in Real Terms, 1960–61 to 1992–93 (in logarithms). Note: base = 1980–81.

Mediclaim insurance scheme covered only 264 000 people. Private health insurance is limited to hospitalization coverage. Only 8 per cent of total health care expenditure is contributed through insurance, about two-thirds is out-of-pocket private expenditure, and the remainder is public expenditure (Chen, 1988).

8.5 POLICY CONCERNS

It is difficult to ascertain whether the presence of private health care provision has had an impact on health outcomes and whether the states where there are more private health care services available exhibit better outcomes than other states. To answer these questions would require observing health status and utilization patterns over a long period of time. However, it was shown above that the utilization of private health care facilities is quite significant, and this undoubtedly has an impact on health status.

There are positive and negative aspects of the significant role of private health care institutions. On the negative side, the growth of the private sector in the country has raised several concerns about quality, cost of care, equity, and efficiency.

One of the major concerns is the scale economies at which private health care services are produced, since they affect cost and quality. In a competitive market, the scale of operations is expected to be optimized by employing the right quantity and mix of services. This optimization should minimize the overall cost of operations and positively affect efficiency. The data reported above, however, showed that hospitals in India have an average capacity of 10 beds. These hospitals may be too small to optimize the mix of resources and minimize costs of production.

Another concern is the sizable out-of-pocket costs incurred by households and expenditure by the private nonhousehold institutional sector. With more than two-thirds of the total health expenditure attributed to these sources, what services are being purchased? Do people get value for money? How do people pay for the costs of catastrophic illnesses? Further research is required to disaggregate expenditure figures and understand the outcomes of services purchased.

The role of private providers in treating illnesses of public health importance has also raised another important concern, particularly in the case of tuberculosis. The disease management practices used by private providers have received strong criticism (Uplekar, 1989a).

8.6   REGULATION OF THE PRIVATE HEALTH SECTOR IN INDIA

8.6.1   Existing regulations

The central and state governments in India have promulgated several pieces of legislation to safeguard the health of their populations. The existing set of regulations related to health care can be broadly divided into three categories:

1. Drug related (for example, the Pharmacy Act, the Drugs and Cosmetics Act, and the Dangerous Drugs Act)
2. Practice related (for example, COPRA, the Indian Medical Council Act, and the Human Organ Transplant Act)
3. Facility related (for example, the NHA, and the Nurses, Midwives and Health Visitors Act).

8.6.2   Assessment of regulations

The assessment of the regulations for this chapter was done in two phases. The first phase sought to determine providers' awareness of the regulations and their assessment of the regulations' effectiveness. The second aimed to understand the implications of these regulations for equity, efficiency, and quality. To address the first issue, a survey (Bhat, 1996) was made of doctors in Ahmedabad.

The results, obtained from written questionnaires and interviews with private doctors in Ahmedabad, are shown in Figure 8.3. It is important to note that, among various regulations, COPRA receives the maximum score. Ninety-three per cent of the respondents indicated their awareness of the main objective of COPRA. One important element of COPRA is that it is applicable throughout India and does not fall within the category of regulations that vary from state to state. The high level of awareness among practising doctors in Ahmedabad about COPRA is indicative of the importance of this piece of legislation affecting private practice in India.

The majority of physicians were also familiar with the Indian Medical Council Act, the MCI Code of Medical Ethics, the Drugs and Cosmetics Act, and the Dangerous

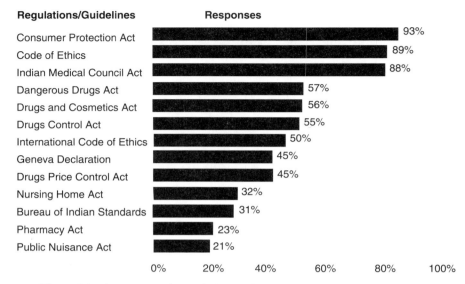

Figure 8.3. Awareness of Regulations Affecting Private Practice in India.

Drugs Act. In comparison, few of the respondents indicated an awareness of the purposes of the eight other Acts listed in Figure 8.3.

Figure 8.4 presents the responses to a question about the effectiveness of these laws and specifically about COPRA. Only 11 per cent of those surveyed believed these laws are ineffective in protecting the interests of patients. About 76 per cent of respondents think that these laws are moderately to highly effective.

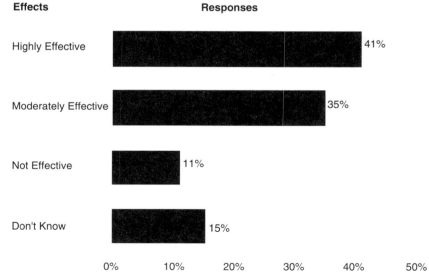

Figure 8.4. Providers' Assessment of the Effectiveness of Regulations in Protecting the Interests of Patients.

Although the respondents think that these laws are effective in protecting patients' interests, they raised doubts about their enforcement. According to the providers, these regulations and policies have been ineffective for the following reasons:

- The implementation and enforcement of rules and regulations have been weak
- The enforcement of different laws has varied from state to state because health is a state responsibility in India
- There has been resistance from various professional groups
- The medical profession has not developed standards and self-regulatory enforcement mechanisms
- Regulations are irrelevant because they have not been updated
- Directing private sector growth is not an important policy objective.

8.7   CASE STUDIES ON REGULATION

Three case studies are presented below to illustrate the impact of regulation on the private health sector.

8.7.1   Case study no. 1: the Consumer Protection Act

The professional bodies governing the medical profession, such as the MCI and medical associations, are an important source of influence to regulate the behavior of private providers. Generally, it is expected that the medical profession will work through self-regulation. However, the associations that were expected to play this role have lost their influence in regulating the behavior of private health care providers because large numbers of physicians are not active members of these associations. And, the active members are not concerned with the guidelines of these associations. As a result, with the growth of the private sector, the prevalence of certain undesirable practices (such as fee-splitting, overprescribing of drugs, inadequate sterilization procedures, employing untrained personnel) has increased.

These undesirable practices have attracted the attention of the consumer movement in India. Recent legislative reforms have now made it possible to bring the medical services provided by the private for-profit sector under COPRA.

8.7.1.1 Overview of the Consumer Protection Act.   COPRA was promulgated in 1986 to protect the interests of consumers through the establishment of consumer councils. The objectives of this Act are to promote and protect the rights of consumers, to provide correct information to protect consumers against unfair trade practices, and to ensure that consumers' interests receive due consideration at appropriate forums. These objectives are promoted by consumer protection councils established at the district, state, and central levels.

The purpose of COPRA is to provide resolution of complaints to aggrieved consumers that is quicker and less costly than the time-consuming and expensive process of civil litigation.

8.7.1.2 Redressal mechanisms. Speedy redressal is provided by quasi-judicial bodies set up at the district, state, and national levels. A complaint under this Act can be filed by an individual consumer or a registered consumer association or the central or state government and a group of consumers with the same interests. A complaint can be lodged if the consumer of services suffers due to a fault, imperfection, shortcoming, or inadequacy in the quality, nature, or manner of performance of a service.

8.7.1.3 Coverage of medical services. COPRA does not include medical services in its list of specified services. Moreover, two categories of services are exempted from the purview of the Act. These are services rendered free of charge or under a contract for personal services. The implication of these two exemptions is that medical services in the public sector are excluded from this Act. Private providers have argued that a service rendered by a medical practitioner is a type of "personal service" and is not the same as a commercial service. Despite these arguments, in two cases filed with the State Commission, the judgment stated that professional services and technical services such as those of surgeons, lawyers, accountants, engineering contractors, etc., are contracts for service, and therefore are covered under COPRA.

8.7.1.4 Response of medical associations. The Indian Medical Association has challenged the judgment in the Supreme Court on the grounds that it cannot include personal contracts within the Act's purview. The association argued that the Act reduces medical services to a seller–buyer relationship. In one of the two above-mentioned cases, the Indian Medical Association and the Qualified Private Medical Practitioners Association appealed to intervene on behalf of the defendants. They argued that the issues raised were of grave concern to members of the association and the medical profession at large. The two associations pleaded that this case should be tried under the Indian Medical Council Act of 1956 because it covers medical doctors and supersedes COPRA. They argued that COPRA does not apply to members of the medical profession. The National Commission did not find merit in their arguments. The Supreme Court recently ruled that COPRA is applicable to any paid medical service.

Another argument that has been made by medical associations and doctors opposing COPRA emanates from fears of misuse of this Act against private providers. This concern does not appear to be legitimate, based on a review of a number of cases filed with the Consumer Disputes and Redressal Commission (CDRC) in Gujarat. Of the total number of cases ruled on since 1991, 71 per cent have been in favor of doctors. Hence, the argument that COPRA's application is unfavorable to private providers is unfounded.

8.7.1.5 Cases of medical negligence. In cases of medical negligence, the onus of proving that the mistake was a result of negligence is on the complainant. In several cases, the complainants faced problems in getting qualified medical practitioners to testify on their behalf, whereas the defendants did not experience any such problem. Getting doctors to testify and explain medical terminology and practice may be a problem in cases of medical negligence. The complainants in the above cases were ultimately unable to furnish qualified witnesses to support their claim.

In most cases, private providers do not make information about diagnoses available to their patients. Patients often do not have information about the medicines they consume. Under these circumstances, the patients are not in a position to build a case with the necessary information and documents as evidence.

8.7.1.6 Effectiveness of the redressal system. The consumer forum is another area that is considered a major obstacle to implementing COPRA. At present, there are about 500 consumer courts in the country. These forums are not adequately staffed and face considerable difficulty because of the lack of necessary infrastructure. The number of cases filed with the consumer forums is growing at a fast rate, yet the forums are not in a position to settle the cases expeditiously. As a result, the number of pending cases is increasing: there are 200 000 cases now pending before these forums. In the medical sector, it was observed that about 50 per cent of the medical cases filed with the CDRC in Gujarat were still pending as of 30 June 1995. This problem may be related to the complexity of medical cases. In the future, it may continue to be difficult for consumer redressal forums to handle the case load pressure and they will become clogged and ineffective.

8.7.1.7 Providers' views. A survey was taken to assess private providers' awareness of the objectives of COPRA and its effectiveness in regulating private medical practice. Sixty-four per cent of respondents believe COPRA is effective in protecting the interests of patients (see Figure 8.5). About 16 per cent of respondents think COPRA is counterproductive to patients' interests, 12 per cent had no opinion about the effectiveness of this legislation, and 8 per cent believe the legislation is ineffective

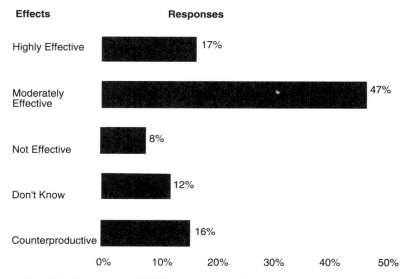

Figure 8.5. Effectiveness of COPRA in Protecting the Interests of Patients: Providers' Assessment.

Table 8.4. Physicians' Perceptions of the Effects of the Consumer Protection Act on Aspects of Private Practice.

Aspects of private practice	Effects				
	Significant increase %	Moderate increase %	No change %	Moderate decrease %	Significant decrease %
Doctors' fee	38	41	19	2	0
Cost of diagnostics	59	32	8	1	0
Prescription of diagnostic procedures	55	36	7	2	0
Prescription of medicines	26	39	29	4	2
Time spent with each patient	19	39	39	3	0
Information given to patients	23	40	33	3	1
Emergency care	27	18	26	12	17
Patient awareness	36	44	16	2	2

Mailed responses = 108, and interviewed = 22, all figures in percentages.

in protecting the interests of patients.

The responses of doctors relating to the effects of COPRA on private medical practice are summarized in Table 8.4. The respondents felt that COPRA has significantly increased doctors' fees: 79 per cent indicated that the effects of this Act have been moderate to high increases in doctors' fees. Another major concern is a potential increase in charges and utilization of diagnostic procedures: 91 per cent believed that the cost and the use of diagnostics have increased. In the providers' view, the increase in the cost of diagnostics and the overuse of diagnostics emerged as major problems of COPRA. About 58 per cent of the respondents thought that the implementation of the Act has increased the amount of time a doctor spends with each patient, whereas 39 per cent of them felt that it has not changed.

Information is an important component that can bridge the communication gap between the doctor and the patient. About 63 per cent of the respondents considered that COPRA led to a moderate to significant increase in information sharing with the patient, whereas 33 per cent felt that the information provided to the patient has not changed.

About 29 per cent of the respondents indicated that the implementation of COPRA has led to a moderate to significant decrease in treating patients in need of immediate care, whereas 45 per cent of the respondents thought that doctors have paid more attention to treating emergency cases. A large number of doctors, about 80 per cent, thought that patient awareness has increased because of COPRA.

In summary, the survey findings revealed that the awareness of the broad objectives of COPRA is high among physicians (over 90 per cent). The majority of them estimated that the Act has had a positive effect on protecting the interests of patients and on providers sharing information. However, it may also have caused overuse of diagnostic tests and drugs and increased doctors' fees.

8.7.1.8 Policy implications. The legislative judgments regarding the applicability of

COPRA to the private medical sector are considered an important policy development. This change has been instrumental in recognizing patients' rights in medical services. It establishes that the patient has the right to question medical treatments and procedures in consumer forums if the provider fails to treat the patient according to standard medical practices and has therefore been negligent.

At the same time, there are apprehensions that private practice will see dramatic changes as a result of the introduction of COPRA. The result of COPRA is expected to be a growing tendency toward practising defensive medicine. Providers are likely to become extremely cautious in treating their patients. The implications of this Act are considered to be an increase in prescribing unnecessary diagnostic tests before treating any patient, resulting in higher costs.

Thus, the desirable consequences of COPRA include increased awareness, increased concern for quality, and additional information for consumers. Among the undesirable consequences could be potential increases in the cost of care, inappropriate care, and a tendency toward practising defensive medicine. Given these consequences, the successful and effective implementation of this Act remains an important question. As with any other policy change, policy-makers are confronted with the problems of minimizing the undesirable consequences of COPRA and, at the same time, removing various constraints to the performance and outcome of this policy in the medical sector.

Major constraints to achieving positive effects through the Act include the lack of a database on the providers and their practice, adequate standards and data about performance, an epidemiological database to determine the risk factors for various disease patterns, a database on risk factors for various diagnostic procedures, an orientation program for doctors, an infrastructure for implementing COPRA, and an effective continuing education program.

8.7.1.9 Making COPRA more effective. There are a number of actions that would make COPRA more effective. First, to overcome the emergence of a defensive medical culture that will cause the cost of care to increase, the medical councils and associations should look at the charge structure for various procedures. Some concerns have already been raised in the Parliament about the fees charged by doctors. The committee of the upper house recommended that doctors notify the MCI of their schedule of fees and that the Council, in turn, make this information available to the public.

Second, the Act has no provision for penalties for people who file false cases. There is apprehension among the providers that the number of false cases will increase and the legislation will be used for harassing providers to extract a settlement. To minimize the misuse of this legislation, it is suggested that there be a screening committee to review cases before they are formally taken up for hearing by the consumer forums. The responsibility of the screening committee would be to categorize cases in such a way that only medical negligence cases posing injury or loss to patients are pursued. Other matters should be referred to the Medical Council.

Third, most doctors feel that the absence of medical professionals from councils is a major drawback of COPRA. This is a result of providers not being involved in enacting COPRA until late in the process. It is argued that nonmedical people make medical judgments when they are not qualified to make an accurate assessment based on the medical evidence. It is suggested that medical people be better represented on the councils, especially in medical negligence cases.

Finally, there should be an orientation program for newly graduated doctors who enter private practice. It is felt that the adoption of service delivery practices is considerably influenced by the environment in which the newly graduated doctors start practising. There should be compulsory continuing education programs. The role of medical councils and associations would be critical in enacting these.

8.7.2   Case study no. 2: Medical Council of India and state medical councils in India

The problem of lack of uniformity in medical education and courses offered by various colleges in India has long been recognized. An Act known as the Indian Medical Degrees Act was passed in 1916 to regulate the granting of titles to persons with Western medical qualifications. In 1956 the Indian government passed the Indian Medical Council Act, whose purpose was to reconstitute the MCI. The 1956 Act was amended in 1964 and 1987 to take care of practical problems in implementing its various provisions and also to grant more powers to the MCI and make it an effective regulatory body.

8.7.2.1 Constitution and composition of the MCI.   The MCI, which meets at least once a year, is an elected body. It is composed of one nominated member from each state, one elected member from each university, one elected member from each state having a medical register, seven members from those enrolled on any of the state medical registers, and eight members nominated by the central government.

8.7.2.2 Functions of the MCI.   The functions of the MCI include giving recognition to medical qualifications granted by medical institutions in India; maintaining the Indian Medical Register; maintaining uniform standards of postgraduate medical education; getting required information on courses of study and examinations from universities and medical institutions in India; and defining a professional code of conduct. However, the Council does not have the power to provide compensation to the aggrieved party even if there is evidence of negligence towards it. Similarly, the MCI cannot order capital punishment in cases of criminal negligence.

8.7.2.3 State medical councils.   State medical councils have been created in various state governments for registering medical practitioners and monitoring and maintaining uniform standards of medical education in the respective states. They are also elected bodies.

8.7.2.4 Role of the councils.   The basic framework of regulatory mechanisms as followed in India to regulate standards of medical education and practice is by empowering the MCI and SMCs. These institutions are supposed to promote self-regulation and compliance.

One of the basic functions of the councils is to maintain a register of providers. However, the councils do not maintain a systematic information database of their registered numbers. For instance, there is no information about the number of providers and their geographic distribution.

The councils have small budgets. The election expenses are borne by the state and central governments. Due to shortage of funds, the elections of the SMCs have been postponed for years in many states. When there have been elections, there have been a number of irregularities in the election process. The councils are vulnerable to political pressures and it is difficult for them to play their regulatory role of maintaining high standards of quality of education and practice.

8.7.2.5 Medical ethics.   The other main activity of the MCI is maintaining and monitoring medical ethics for practising doctors. All medical applicants at the time of registration are bound by the Geneva declaration accepted by the General Assembly of the World Medical Association in London on 12 October 1949. This declaration provides a code of professional conduct.

The MCI has produced a list of the types of professional misconduct that can be presented to the Council for disciplinary action. The Council punishes physicians by removing their names from the register entirely or for a specified period.

The MCI's list of professional offenses and misconduct is not complete, however, as it is not exhaustive, nor does it identify punishments. In cases of misconduct, the Council must deliberate and decide on the action to be taken against the medical practitioner.

There have been few instances of medical councils intervening and initiating disciplinary action against members of their profession even when there is a formal complaint of negligence. Informal discussions with one of the council members revealed that not many councils have suspended the registration of any member even though many complaints are received by the Council. In the case of one council, inquiry was initiated in only three cases and, in those, no disciplinary action has been taken.

At the same time, consumer courts have been receiving numerous complaints against registered members of the MCI. In most cases, a copy of the complaint is also forwarded to the councils. Some of the regulations regarding punishment under the Indian Medical Council Act have become outdated.

8.7.2.6 The role of government.   The role of government in overseeing the councils is quite limited. Officials of the central or state government will intervene only if they have reason to believe that the councils are not following any of the provisions of this Act; they may refer the complaint to the Commission of Inquiry, which is composed of two people appointed by the central government and one by the MCI. The Commission of Inquiry makes recommendations if it finds the council guilty of the charges against it or if the council has taken improper actions.

8.7.2.7 Future directions.   In summary, the performance of the MCI and SMCs as regulators has been less than impressive in India. They have failed to regulate the medical profession and to set adequate standards to safeguard the interest of patients, particularly in the area of medical practice. As a first step, the role of regulating education should be separated from the role of regulating medical practice. This would require a separate commission to establish adequate standards and ensure their implementation. The character of medical care in India has changed drastically and these changes need to be addressed by the MCI. In order to do so, however, the basic structure and financing of the MCI have to be strengthened to make it an effective organization.

8.7.3   Case study no. 3: the Nursing Home Act

Nursing homes, which are small private hospitals and dispensaries in India, constitute an important component of the private health care delivery system. These institutions provide both inpatient and outpatient services in general medicine or specialty care to patients of all age groups. Nursing homes in India have experienced rapid growth.

The NHA for the state of Maharashtra defines a nursing home as any premise used or intended to be used for the reception of persons suffering from any sickness, injury, or infirmity and the provision of treatment and nursing for them. It includes maternity homes. These facilities usually have a capacity of fewer than 25 beds and do not generally have the basic facilities required of a full-service hospital. Nursing homes in India are primarily owned by a doctor or a group of doctors.

Nursing homes in India have grown without regulation except in two states, Maharashtra and Delhi. In these two states, the Bombay NHA and the Delhi NHA regulate the registration of nursing homes.

8.7.3.1 Registration and renewal of registration.   The NHAs in Maharashtra and Delhi require that any person interested in starting a nursing home apply for registration with the local supervising authority (municipality or district board). A similar application is also submitted each year to the local supervising authority for renewal of such registration.

8.7.3.2 Inspection of nursing homes.   The second important provision is that health officers of the local supervising authority may enter and inspect a registered nursing home. They can inspect any records required by the provisions of the Act.

8.7.3.3 Implementation of NHAs.   The local supervising authorities in these two states have failed to implement the broad provisions of the NHA. As a result, these laws have been ineffective in regulating the growth and development of nursing homes in Maharashtra and Delhi.

First, there are problems with registration. In a survey of 65 stratified randomly selected nursing homes in Delhi, only 22 per cent were registered under the Delhi NHA. It was also found that only 130 of approximately 1200 nursing homes in Delhi are registered with one of the local supervising authorities. Since the situation in Maharashtra is no different, the result is that a large number of such facilities are operating in these two states without registration.

Second, inspection of nursing homes is rare. For example, the municipal corporation in Bombay admitted during hearings that, in several wards of the city, officials had neither visited any nursing home nor taken action against any nursing home for several years.

Third, instances of cancellation of registration of nursing homes are infrequent in these states. This reflects the difficulties in implementing these laws. Many surveys indicate that large numbers of nursing homes in these states are in a deplorable condition. In Bombay, a study has shown that 63 per cent of the hospitals were located in residential premises, and 12.5 per cent were run from sheds that had inadequate roofs. Only 8 per cent functioned in independent buildings. The study further showed that 50 per cent of the hospitals were located in poorly maintained buildings or were dilapidated.

The Nandraj (1994) study showed that several hospitals and nursing homes that were surveyed did not have operating rooms. Those that did, did not meet adequate standards: they had leaks, peeling paint, no scrubbing room, or no emergency support services. The Yesudian (1994) study found that private nursing homes and clinics did not have adequate medical equipment. The equipment on hand was unreliable, poorly maintained, and improperly operated.

8.7.3.4 Reforms required. The NHAs do not specify minimum standards for nursing homes. Since nursing home legislation does not normally specify standards, such standards could be established by the medical associations or the MCI. The standard-setting agency should then be empowered to monitor those standards.

The process of registration and renewal of nursing home registration should also be tightened and strictly enforced. The local supervising authorities should be made responsible for registration and renewal of registration. However, since the local authorities do not have the capacity to perform inspection, it should be done by the standard-setting agency proposed above. Some kind of accreditation system should be put in place and all nursing homes should be regularly surveyed.

In Bombay and Delhi, the growth of nursing homes has been haphazard. Most of the homes are concentrated in a few areas. The local supervising agencies have not planned the distribution of nursing homes. The proper distribution of nursing homes could be controlled through registration.

Most of the nursing homes have adopted medical technology. In a survey of nursing homes in Delhi, 75 per cent had ultrasound equipment and 26 per cent had scans. At the time of registration and renewal, the NHAs are not required to inform the local supervising authority about what equipment they have. There needs to be some system of equitable distribution of medical technologies.

The NHAs do not specify what information the nursing homes should submit to the local supervising authority, except records of deaths and births. Data on disease patterns could be submitted to local supervising authorities for policy decisions regarding public health issues.

The existing regulations are outdated. For example, one penalty clause has a fine of only Rs. 100 (in the first quarter of 1996, Rs. 100 = US $2.85). To ensure better compliance, particularly in the area of registration and renewal of registration, the penalties should be much higher.

The Ministry of Health in India should take a broad view of the regulation of nursing homes in India and lay down basic policy guidelines for all states. The state of Karnataka has already appointed a high-powered committee to consider the regulation of nursing homes, hospitals, and diagnostic centers. The central government should urge other states to evolve their own guidelines in order to monitor and control the growth and development of nursing homes in India.

8.8   CONCLUSION

The private sector is a significant part of the Indian health care system in terms of facilities, human resources, and expenditure. It continues to grow at a rapid pace. Yet, as the three case studies show, the mechanisms for monitoring and regulating the private sector have not kept pace. Certain Acts have been passed but have not been adequately implemented. Other areas require regulation. The challenge for the future will be to develop the regulatory mechanisms that will ensure quality and efficiency in the delivery of health services by the private health sector.

Another policy concern is the large role played by private sector providers in treating many illnesses of public health importance, such as diarrhea, respiratory infection, and tuberculosis. How can these be linked with existing major public sector efforts to treat and prevent such health problems? Finding mechanisms to harness the energies of the private sector to support public sector efforts to promote national health objectives will be another challenge in the coming years.

REFERENCES

Bhat, R. (1993). The private/public mix in health care in India. *Health Policy and Planning*, **8**(1), 43–56.

Bhat, R. (1996). Regulating the private health care sector: the case of the Indian Consumer Protection Act. *Health Policy and Planning*, **11**(3), 265–279.

Central Bureau of Health Intelligence (1985 and 1988). *Directory of Hospitals in India*. New Delhi: Ministry of Health and Family Welfare, Government of India.

Chatterjee, M. (1988). *Implementing Health Policy*. New Delhi: Centre for Policy Research.

Chen, L. (1988). Health policy responses: an approach derived from China and India experiences. In: Bell, D. E., Reich, M. R. (Eds). *Health, Nutrition, and Economic Crises*. Dover, MA: Auburn House Publishing Company, 279–305.

de Ferranti, D. (1985). *Paying for Health Services in Developing Countries: An Overview*. World Bank Staff Working Paper No. 721. Washington, DC: World Bank.

Duggal, R., Amin, S. (1989). *Cost of Health Care: A Household Survey in an Indian District*. Bombay: Foundation for Research in Community Health.

Jesani, A., Anantharam, S. (1989). *Private Sector and Privatisation in the Health Care Services*. Bombay: Foundation for Research in Community Health.

Nandraj, S. (1994). Beyond the law and the Lord: quality of private health care. *Economic and Political Weekly*, July 2, 1994, 1680–1685.

Satia, J. K., Deodhar, N. (1993). Hospital costs and financing in Maharashtra: a case study. In: Berman, P., Khan, M. (Eds). *Paying for India's Health Care*. New Delhi: Sage Publications.

Satia, J. K., Giridhar, G., Pandey, I., Dholakia, B., Dholakia, R. (1987). *Study of Health Care Financing in India.* Ahmedabad: Indian Institute of Management.

Uplekar, M. (1989a). *Implications of Prescribing Patterns in Private Doctors in the Treatment of Pulmonary Tuberculosis in Bombay, India.* Research Paper No. 41. Takemi Program in International Health. Cambridge: Harvard School of Public Health.

Uplekar, M. (1989b). *Private Doctors and Public Health: The Case of Leprosy in Bombay.* Research Paper No. 40. Takemi Program in International Health. Cambridge: Harvard School of Public Health.

Vishwanathan, H., Rohde, J. (1990). *Diarrhoea in Rural India: A Nation-wide Study of Mothers and Practitioners.* New Delhi: Vision Books.

Yesudian, C. (1990). *Utilization Pattern of Health Services and its Implications for Urban Health Policy.* Takemi Program in International Health. Cambridge: Harvard School of Public Health. Draft.

Yesudian, C. (1994). The nature of private sector health services in Bombay. *Health Policy and Planning,* **9**(1), 72–80.

9

Private Health Sector Performance and Regulation in the Philippines

ALEJANDRO HERRIN

School of Economics, University of the Philippines

9.1 INTRODUCTION

The private sector in the Philippines is seen not only as an initiator but also as a prime mover of development. This sector has traditionally dominated economic activities and is a major provider and financier of such social services as education and health. However, the government continues to play a significant role in the economy not only as a provider and financier but also as a regulator of economic and social activities.

This chapter provides a brief profile of the private health sector in the Philippines and then describes the factors affecting its development. Emphasis is placed on the role of the government in promoting private health sector development.

9.2 PROFILE OF THE PRIVATE HEALTH SECTOR

The private health sector can be described from the standpoints of health care financing, delivery, and utilization.

9.2.1 *Financing*

In 1991, national health care expenditure in the Philippines totaled 29.5 billion pesos, representing about 2.3 per cent of gross national product (GNP). Major sources of financing included government (national and local), social insurance (Medicare and Employees Compensation), household out-of-pocket payments, health maintenance organizations (HMOs), and private health insurance (see Table 9.1). Data on enterprise-based and community-based financing are not yet available. Research is continuing to obtain estimates of health expenditures from these sources.

Of the total documented health expenditure, 44 per cent was financed by the government: 39 per cent by the national government and 5 per cent by local governments (see Table 9.2). The social insurance programs, namely the Medicare

Private Health Sector Growth in Asia: Issues and Implications. Edited by W. Newbrander.
© 1997 John Wiley & Sons, Ltd.

Table 9.1. National Health Account Expenditures in Thousands of Pesos, 1991.

Uses of funds	Sources of funds						Total by use of funds
	Government		Social insurance		Private		
	National	Local	Medicare	Employees compensation	Out-of-pocket	Private insurance and HMOs	
Personal health care	7 130 711	379 463	1 732 475	90 369	11 316 292	592 054	21 241 364
Public health care	2 836 244	1 000 308	—	—	—	—	3 836 552
Others	1 671 763	—	1 380 120	306 992	—	1 104 133	4 463 008
Total	11 638 718	1 379 771	3 112 595	397 361	11 316 292	1 696 187	29 540 924

Data on enterprise-based and community-based financing are not yet available. (Estimates as of November, 1994.)
Source: Racelis and Herrin (1994).

Table 9.2. Percentage Distribution of National Health Account Expenditures, 1991.

Uses of funds	Sources of funds						Total by use of funds
	Government		Social insurance		Private		
	National	Local	Medicare	Employees compensation	Out-of-pocket	Private insurance and HMOs	
Personal health care	24.1	1.3	5.9	0.3	38.3	2.0	71.9
Public health care	9.6	3.4	0.0	0.0	0.0	0.0	13.0
Others	5.7	0.0	4.7	1.0	0.0	3.7	15.1
Total	39.4	4.7	10.6	1.3	38.3	5.7	100.0

Program and the Employees Compensation Program, financed about 12 per cent of total health expenditure. The remainder (44 per cent) was financed by the private sector: 38 per cent from out-of pocket payments by households and 6 per cent by private insurance and HMOs.

9.2.2 Delivery

9.2.2.1 Health facilities.   Health services are offered by different types of private and government providers in the Philippines.[1] Health facilities operated by the government provide preventive, curative, and rehabilitative services, while those operated by the private sector tend to focus on direct personal, mainly curative, care. Government health facilities include hospitals of various categories (primary, secondary, and tertiary) and primary health care facilities consisting of *barangay* (village) health stations and rural health units. Private health facilities consist of hospitals owned and managed by single proprietors, corporations, or charitable organizations. In addition, an undetermined number of clinics are owned and operated by private physicians.

Table 9.3 and Figure 9.1 illustrate the growth of hospitals and hospital beds during the 23-year period from 1970 to 1993. The number of hospitals and hospital beds owned by the private sector grew rapidly in the 1970s and declined slowly in the 1990s. In contrast, the number of hospitals and hospital beds owned by the government continued to grow up to 1990; thereafter these too began to decline. It is not yet clear what factors were responsible for these trends. However, as will be described later, the growth of private hospitals in the 1970s was facilitated by the introduction of Medicare, while their decline in the 1980s was related to economic difficulties during that period.

In 1993, there were 1632 hospitals of various categories, of which 67 per cent were private hospitals. However, of the total 71 865 beds, only half were private. Thus private hospitals, while more numerous, tend to have smaller bed numbers than government hospitals.

Data on the distribution of hospitals and hospital beds by category reveal that 83 per cent of primary hospitals (and 82 per cent of hospital beds) are private. Among secondary hospitals, the private sector accounted for 56 per cent of the total number and 52 per cent of total beds. Finally, among tertiary hospitals, the private sector accounted for 57 per cent of all hospitals but only 40 per cent of the hospital beds.

There is an uneven geographical distribution of hospital beds in each category. The tertiary hospital beds, however, are much more unevenly distributed, with a very high concentration of both public and private beds in Metro Manila relative to the rest of the regions.

9.2.2.2 Health providers.   Very little information exists about the number and distribution of health providers outside of those employed in the government. A study undertaken in 1990 was the first systematic study that attempted to estimate the number of four different types of health providers from various data sources. The

---

[1]The producers of health inputs (such as the health professional education market, the drug manufacturing industry, and the producers of medical equipment and supplies) are nearly all private.

Table 9.3. Public and Private Hospitals and Beds, Number and Percentage.

| Year | Number of hospitals | | | | | Bed capacity | | | | | Beds per 10 000 population |
| | Total | Public | | Private | | Total | Public | | Private | | |
		No.	%	No.	%		No.	%	No.	%	
1970	650	220	34	430	66	40 271	19 725	49	20 546	51	10.9
1980	1607	413	26	1194	74	81 796	39 445	48	42 351	52	13.0
1990	1733	598	35	1135	65	87 133	49 273	57	37 860	43	12.9
1993	1632	537	33	1095	67	71 865	35 629	50	36 236	50	10.7

Source: National Statistical Coordination Board, *1994 Philippine Statistical Yearbook.*

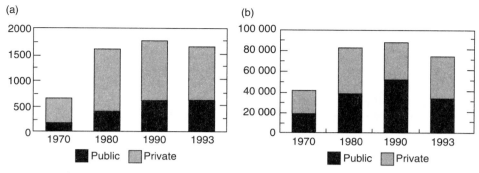

Figure 9.1. Number of (a) Hospitals and (b) Hospital Beds, 1970–93.

Table 9.4. Number of Employed Health Staff in the Public and Private Sectors, 1987.

| | Staff category | | | |
Institution	Physician	Nurses	Midwives	Dentists
Public sector				
Department of Health				
Regional, provincial, and health officers	455	397	118	95
Rural health units	2086	2711	10 177	1019
Hospitals	4371	6340	392	312
Subtotal	6912	9448	10 687	1426
Other government departments				
Department of Education	123	1047	—	577
Department of Local Government	296	546	136	484
Department of National Defense	288	699	231	331
Office of the President	40	103	47	—
Subtotal	747	2395	414	1392
Total	7659	11 843	11 101	2818
Percentage of total employees	42%	53%	76%	33%
Private sector	10 634	10 570	3510	5780
Percentage of total employees	58%	47%	24%	67%
Total employees	18 293	22 413	14 611	8598
Professional Association's estimate of total number of practitioners	18 500	50 000	—	10 000

Source: Reyes and Picazo (1990).

results shown in Table 9.4 indicate that the private sector employed 58 per cent of the physicians, 47 per cent of the nurses, 24 per cent of the midwives, and 67 per cent of the dentists.

A recent study that was based on a sample of the 1990 census and designed to determine the regional distribution and place of work of selected health professionals (see Solon *et al.*, 1995) reveals the following:[2]

---

[2]The study obtained only sample frequencies rather than a national estimate of the total number of health professionals by specific categories.

- Eighty-seven per cent of physicians work in hospitals (65 per cent in private and 22 per cent in public hospitals), while the rest work in schools, industrial establishments, and other workplaces. A large majority (93 per cent) work in urban areas. Moreover, 64 per cent of all physicians work in Metro Manila and the adjacent regions of Southern Tagalog and Central Luzon
- Seventy-four per cent of dentists practise in private hospitals, clinics, and laboratories, 10 per cent in public facilities, 3 per cent in schools, and the rest in industrial establishments and other workplaces. As many as 91 per cent work in urban areas. Moreover, 71 per cent are found in Metro Manila, Southern Tagalog, and Central Luzon
- Seventy-eight per cent of nurses work in hospitals, clinics, and laboratories (49 per cent in private facilities and 29 per cent in public facilities), while the rest work in schools, industrial establishments, and other workplaces. Like other health professionals, nurses are unevenly distributed, with 52 per cent found in Metro Manila, Southern Tagalog, and Central Luzon
- Seventy-seven per cent of midwives work in hospital facilities (42 per cent in private facilities and 35 per cent in public facilities). In contrast to other health professionals, midwives are more evenly distributed across the country, with only 46 per cent found in Metro Manila, Southern Tagalog, and Central Luzon.

As for the other categories of health providers, such as medical technologists, sanitary inspectors, nutritionists/dietitians, and pharmacists, little is known about their numbers and geographic distribution except those who are employed by the Department of Health (DOH).

In addition to medical personnel, services are provided by the traditional health sector, including the *herbolarios* and *hilots*. Herbolarios are general practitioners of traditional medicine. Hilots are traditional birth attendants or traditional midwives. There is no information regarding their numbers and distribution, although there is probably at least one hilot in each of the more than 40 000 villages in the Philippines. Hilots still attend to a very large proportion of total births (52 per cent), as revealed by the *1993 National Safe Motherhood Survey* (National Statistics Office, 1994b). In 1975 the DOH started training hilots in maternal and child health care, herbal medicine, and information, education, and communication activities. By 1990 the DOH reported that some 33 500 hilots had undergone such training (DOH, as reported in Herrin *et al.*, 1992).

9.2.3 Utilization

Another way of looking at the role of the private health sector is to assess to what extent private health sector facilities, personnel, or services are used by the population. A few national surveys have obtained data on utilization both of health facilities and of some specific services. Not all data, however, distinguish whether the facilities or personnel visited for consultation or service are private or public. The few available data are briefly described below.

Table 9.5 and Figure 9.2 show the percentage of households that have used specific health facilities during the 12 months prior to the 1987 National Health Survey.

Table 9.5. Percentage of Households That Have Used Selected Health Facilities, by Income Class, 1987.

Income class (in pesos)	Distribution of households	Public hospital	Private hospital/clinic	Rural health unit	Barangay health station
Philippines	100.0	32.2	34.1	32.6	36.2
Under 10 000	19.2	27.6	19.4	34.4	40.6
10 000–14 999	18.4	31.6	25.4	38.7	42.2
15 000–19 999	15.4	34.1	31.2	36.4	41.2
20 000–29 999	17.2	35.8	36.9	34.2	36.9
30 000–39 999	10.1	34.8	44.9	29.4	31.6
40 000–59 999	8.9	32.7	47.8	26.1	28.2
60 000 and over	10.6	30.1	54.3	19.4	21.0

Source: Department of Health, National Health Survey (1987).

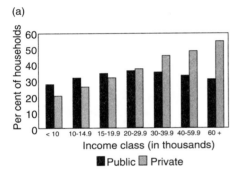

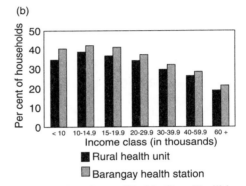

Figure 9.2. Household Use of (a) Hospitals and (b) Public Primary Health Care Facilities, 1987.

Each household was asked whether any member of the household visited a specific facility. A household may use several facilities, both public and private, during the year. The data show that about a third of households have visited each of the following facilities: government hospital, private hospital/clinic, rural health unit, and barangay health station.

A household's use of private hospitals generally increases with income, while a household's use of government primary care facilities declines with income. The household's use of government hospitals remains more or less the same across income groups at around 30 per cent. Similar data obtained by the 1992 National Health Survey show that, during that year, the percentages of households that availed themselves of health services at government hospitals, rural health units, barangay health stations, and private hospitals and clinics were 23, 30, 22, and 26, respectively. As in the previous data, a household can use several facilities during the year.

Table 9.6 shows that among the members of the households in the 1987 National Health Survey who were reported to be ill and who sought medical consultation, 52 per cent went to a public health facility, while 41 per cent went to a private hospital

Table 9.6. Percentage of the Population Seeking Treatment for Illness, by Place of Treatment and Type of Medical Attendant, 1987.

Place of consultation	Percentage
Public sector	52.4
Goverment hospital	19.8
Rural health unit	19.9
Puericulture center	1.0
Barangay health station	11.7
Private sector	41.1
Private hospital	18.3
Private clinic	22.8
Home	6.5
Type of medical attendant	
Government physician	34.0
Private physician	42.6
Nurse	6.6
Midwife	16.8

Percentages reflect the number of people who reported sick during the 7 days prior to the survey who sought treatment for that illness.
Source: Department of Health, National Health Survey (1987).

or clinic. A small percentage were visited at home. In terms of the type of medical attendant, 43 per cent went to a private physician, while about a third went to a government physician, and about a quarter went to a nurse or a midwife.

With respect to dental care, data from the 1992 National Health Survey show that 40 per cent of the households surveyed have members who sought consultation for dental problems. Of these, 44 per cent went to a private dentist, 37 per cent went to government dentists, either at a government hospital or at rural health units, and 10 per cent went to school-based dentists. It is not clear, however, whether these school dentists worked in public or private schools.

While the national data show that the total population used both public and private facilities and personnel roughly equally, data on the poorest segment of the population (the bottom 30 per cent of the income distribution)[3] show that they overwhelmingly use public facilities or personnel either for general consultation, or for specific services such as prenatal care or child immunization. However, hilots predominantly attend to deliveries in the mother's home (Herrin and Racelis, 1994).

More recent data from the 1993 National Safe Motherhood Survey (National Statistics Office, 1994b) show that a large proportion (77 per cent) of prenatal visits were made to public facilities, while 70 per cent of births took place at home, 52 per cent with the assistance of hilots. Data from the 1993 National Demographic Survey (National Statistics Office, 1994a) show that about 71 per cent of modern family planning supplies were obtained from public health facilities, while the private health sector accounted for only 26 per cent.

---

[3]The 1992 Socio-Economic Survey of Special Groups of Families.

In sum, what the data (albeit incomplete) suggest is that there is a market for both public and private sector health services and that these vary by specific type of service. Most primary care services are obtained from government primary health care facilities; hospital care is obtained in private hospitals by higher-income groups; and a large proportion of deliveries are still attended by hilots, representing the traditional private sector (although a number of these hilots have had training from the DOH).

9.3 THE DEVELOPMENT OF THE PRIVATE HEALTH CARE SECTOR

The development of the private health sector is due to a number of interacting factors. These factors include the growth of household incomes, the inadequacies of the public health sector, and the effects of various government policies on the operation of different health care markets. Although it is not possible to analyze the quantitative effects of these factors due to data limitations, the general economic environment and major government policies that are thought to have influenced the development of the private health sector in the past 20 years are described in this section.

9.3.1 General economic environment

In the past two decades, the performance of the Philippine economy has not kept pace with those of neighboring countries. While real GNP grew at an average rate of 6.2 per cent in the 1970s, the average growth rate fell to 1.7 per cent in the 1980s. In fact, the economy contracted in 1984 and 1985. The slow economic growth, combined with continued rapid population growth, resulted in slow growth in per capita income. The economy has yet to recover from the sharp drop in per capita income in 1984 and 1985.

The decline in per capita income in the mid-1980s and the slow economic recovery is reflected in continued high rates of poverty.[4] The slow growth in per capita income and high poverty rates meant a correspondingly slow growth in the capacity of the population to pay for health-promoting goods and services, including health care. This, in turn, would tend to slow down the growth of the private health sector.

Coupled with the slow economic growth is the slow structural transformation of the economy. The share of employment in the manufacturing sector and the other industrial sectors has barely changed since the 1950s. Data from 1970 to 1994 show that the employed labor force in both manufacturing and other industries was about 16 per cent in 1970, about the same as in 1994. Among other factors, this slow structural transformation has hindered the more rapid expansion of social insurance and employer-based financing systems that could have expanded the demand for private health services.

---

[4]The povery rate was estimated by the National Economic and Development Authority at 44.2 per cent in 1985, 40.2 per cent in 1988, and 39.2 per cent in 1991. A recent preliminary estimate showed that the poverty rate in 1994 was 35.7 per cent (National Statistical Coordination Board, *Poverty Statistics: 1991 Revised Estimates and 1994 Preliminary Estimates*, November 1995). Although this represented an improvement over the 1991 figure, this still meant that there were 4.6 million families below the poverty threshold in 1994. A revised estimate for 1991 is 39.9 per cent.

9.3.2   Government policies affecting the supply of health services

Government policies influence the operation of the private health sector either through the supply side (by affecting the growth of health inputs, such as health providers and health facilities) or through the demand side (by affecting the growth of people's purchasing power through the development of various health care financing systems).

9.3.2.1 Supply of health providers.   A factor facilitating the growth of the private health sector is the availability of health providers, produced by a predominantly private professional education sector. Schools for health professionals (physicians, nurses, midwives, and dentists), which, like all other schools, are licensed by the government, have increased over the years, resulting in the growth of enrollment and new entrants into the health profession. A recent study showed that in 1975 there were only 10 medical schools, 73 nursing schools, and seven dentistry schools in the country. By 1988, their numbers had risen to 25, 126, and 16, respectively. Moreover, in 1988, there were 113 schools of midwifery (Reyes and Picazo, 1990).

These schools are producing a large group of health professionals. In 1993, for example, those who passed the board examinations numbered 2302 (medicine), 24 880 (nursing), and 1148 (dentistry). During the period 1988 to 1991, the total numbers who passed the board examinations were 9895 (medicine), 40 392 (nursing), and 7422 (dentistry). However, a recent study revealed that during the same period, 1988–91, a total of 1305 physicians, 10 393 nurses, and 801 dentists were lost through emigration and temporary overseas employment. Of those lost to other countries, a large majority of the physicians and dentists (96 and 88 per cent, respectively) were lost through emigration, while 82 per cent of nurses were lost through temporary overseas employment (Rodriguez *et al.*, 1993).

Although it encourages private sector participation in professional education, the government — through the Department of Education, Culture, and Sports — regulates the admission and curricular requirements of medical, nursing, dental, and other schools for health professionals, purportedly to maintain standards of quality. Moreover, the Professional Regulation Commission is in charge of the licensing examinations. With respect to physicians, the professional medical associations, which are private institutions, set up their own boards to certify specialists.

In sum, despite government regulations and professional certification requirements, the predominantly private professional education sector was relatively free to expand the supply of health providers in response to increasing domestic and foreign demand.

9.3.2.2 Health care facilities.   Several government regulations affect the growth and viability of private hospitals.[5] The first is the licensure of hospitals. No hospital, whether public or private, may operate without a license issued by the Bureau of Licensing and Regulation of the DOH. As a requirement for licensing, all hospitals

---

[5] While hospitals are closely regulated, there is no regulatory framework governing the establishment of private outpatient clinics (Solon *et al.*, 1995). The only requirement seems to be a business license required by local government units. There is no information regarding the number of such clinics nor their locations.

must meet certain prescribed technical standards in personnel, equipment, and physical facilities depending on the type of hospital (for example, primary, secondary, tertiary, or training or nontraining).

Requirements for standards are often justified as necessary for assuring quality of health care. However, very strict standards may limit hospital expansion by increasing the cost of establishing a new hospital. In view of the rapid growth of both public and private hospitals, it appears that licensing standards as currently set — or enforced — were not a major constraint to hospital growth. Alternatively, these constraints may have been negated by powerful economic forces.

In addition to requiring licensure and technical standards, the government has instituted rules that affect the revenues of private hospitals (Griffin et al., 1994). These include requiring private hospitals to set aside at least 10 per cent of their authorized bed capacity for charity patients; requiring private hospitals to treat emergency patients even when they are unable to pay their medical bills (in practice this provision takes the form of preventing private hospitals from requiring a money deposit from a patient being treated for an emergency); and taxation of income of for-profit hospitals at the same rate as other corporate institutions (usually 35 per cent of net income).[6]

There is little information regarding the impact of these requirements on the viability and growth of the private hospitals. To compensate for those who are unable to pay for hospital stays and emergency treatments, there is always the possibility of shifting the extra burden of financing to the paying patients. As for the taxation of income, it has been observed that this has created incentives to modify the organization of hospitals or their tax status in order to avoid the income tax (for example, establishing the hospital as a teaching school of nursing or midwifery to take advantage of the different tax status of educational institutions).

9.3.2.3 Availability of credit for financing the construction of private hospitals. While government regulation of health providers and facilities might have a constraining effect on the expansion of the private sector, the government has, in fact, promoted the growth of the private health sector and encouraged the dispersal of health facilities across the country by providing access to financial capital. From an economy-wide perspective, this is nothing very special, since the government has been providing easy access to credit and tax incentives to the other sectors of the economy, particularly the manufacturing sector.

The following is a brief summary of the history of the government's lending program to private hospitals (Griffin et al., 1994). From 1966 to 1969, the Development Bank of the Philippines embarked on a substantial lending program for hospitals. Loans were granted to members of the medical profession or to

---

[6]A recent study suggested that while the government does have a small budget to pay for charity patients in private hospitals who do not have access to a public hospital, and that private hospitals are allowed by law to claim income tax deductions for services rendered to emergency patients who are unable to pay their medical bills, these provisions have rarely been realized, at least according to the hospital owners who were interviewed in the study (Griffin et al., 1994).

corporations organized predominantly by medical practitioners for the establishment of new, and improvement of existing, hospitals and medical clinics.

The Medical Care Act of 1969 provided further impetus to lending by providing that hospitals be given priority by government financing institutions, especially in the rural areas where there were no existing government or private hospitals as determined by the Philippine Medical Care Commission. In October 1978, this was supplemented by a special financing program for hospitals with bed capacities of 100 beds and below in areas that had been identified as "bed deficient".

The economic crisis experienced in the mid-1980s, however, led not only to severe fund shortages on the part of financing institutions but also to business failures. Many hospitals that overborrowed or were poorly managed failed and had to close down. This reinforced decisions to eliminate loan windows on the industry. After 1986, only the Social Security System (SSS) was left with a concessional loan window devoted to hospital development. Thus, at present, hospitals are left to compete with other industries in the commercial loan market. These developments partly explain the slow growth of the private hospital sector in the 1980s.

9.3.3   Government policies affecting the demand for health services

In addition to policies affecting the supply side, the growth of the private health sector has been promoted by government intervention on the demand side, mainly through the development of social insurance and through requirements for health service provision by employers.

9.3.3.1 Medicare. The Medicare Program is a compulsory health insurance program established by law in 1969 and implemented in 1972 with the creation of the Philippine Medical Care Commission. As of 1991, Medicare was estimated to have covered about 26 million members and dependants representing 42 per cent of the total population (Patao and Jeffers, 1994). The Medicare Program provides for inpatient benefits through accredited public and private hospitals.

As Table 9.1 shows, in 1991 the benefits paid by Medicare totaled 3.1 billion pesos. In spite of its 20-year history, this program was financing only 11 per cent of total expenditures. Nonetheless, the Medicare Program has helped widen access to health services by giving its members and their dependants financial support to pay for unpredictable and large hospitalization costs. The increase in demand for health services arising from this funding support is believed to have given impetus to the expansion of the private hospital sector after 1972.

The potential impact of Medicare on the growth of the private sector, however, has been constrained by a number of factors. One factor is the low and declining support value of Medicare (the proportion of the total medical bill paid for by the insurance). Originally designed with a support value of 70 per cent in 1972, its actual support value dropped to only 32 per cent in 1989 before it was adjusted during that year. The support value is currently believed to be around 50 per cent, which means that the patient effectively copays 50 per cent of the total medical bill. A low support value limits the greater use of health services by beneficiaries who are unable to afford this large copayment.

A second factor that has limited the impact of Medicare is related to the slow structural transformation of the economy mentioned earlier. This factor prevented a rapid increase in the number of beneficiaries from the organized employed sector that could be efficiently covered by the program. A third reason is the lack of strong efforts by the Medicare Program, through the SSS, to compel firms to enroll their employees in Medicare.

9.3.3.2 Employees Compensation Program. In addition to the Medicare Program, the government also mandates employers to provide medical and disability benefits through the Employees Compensation Program. The Employees Compensation Program was established in 1975 and administered by the Employees Compensation Commission, which is in turn directly supervised by the Department of Labor and Employment (DOLE). As Table 9.2 shows, the Employees Compensation Program financed only a minor portion (1.3 per cent) of total health expenditure in 1991; hence, it has not been a major factor in expanding demand for health care. Part of the reason for its minor role in financing is the difficulty of establishing whether the employee's illness or disability was work related.

9.3.3.3 Labor Code provisions. The government, through the Labor Code, also mandates employers to provide medical services to their employees. The Labor Code specifies the minimal medical and dental service obligations of employers. Specific requirements, ranging from providing first aid to provisions for a company clinic with medical staff, are set according to the number of employees and the hazards involved in the work. Employer responses have varied, including directly providing the services in company-based facilities. For example, some mining companies and large agricultural plantations have set up hospitals for their employees; other employers have enrolled their employees in private group insurance or in HMOs.

Information is lacking regarding the health expenditures that employers incur on behalf of their employees. The DOLE is supposed to monitor employers' compliance with the provisions of the Labor Code. However, the DOLE claims that, due to lack of personnel, it is unable to monitor the thousands of enterprises effectively.

9.3.3.4 Private insurance. Data for 1987 showed that there were 103 companies offering health and accident insurance in the country: 93 nonlife and 10 life insurance (Rodriguez *et al.*, 1993). The regulation of health insurance companies is carried out by the Office of the Insurance Commissioner. The numerous requirements and restrictions imposed on insurance companies are aimed at minimizing the chance of nonperformance on contracts or default by the insurer. Such requirements include margin-of-solvency requirements, limits on investments, limits on risks taken, reserve requirements, and examination and licensing of insurance agents. These requirements and restrictions increase the cost of insurance, which then tends to limit the role of private insurance in total health care financing and, consequently, in private health sector expansion.

9.3.3.5 Health maintenance organizations. Health maintenance organizations are relatively new in the Philippines. As of 1993, there were 17 HMOs operating in the

Philippines, mostly investor-based (the others include employer-based and community-based HMOs). Investor-based HMO companies target corporate clients, taking advantage of government requirements for providing medical services to their employees. It is not clear whether employer-based health benefits through HMOs represent additional benefits over previously provided benefits or simply a shift in the manner of financing employer-based benefits. Since HMOs are relatively new, they do not yet fall under any government agency's regulatory umbrella. The Association of HMOs has favored self-regulation.

9.3.3.6 Community financing schemes. A growing number of community-based health care financing mechanisms have been identified through contests sponsored by the Health and Management Information Project of the DOH and the German Agency for Technical Cooperation. In two contests, cash prizes were given to community-based institutions that demonstrated innovativeness, quality of care, effectiveness of programs, efficiency, equity, and sustainability. The contests help identify institutions that otherwise would not be known because there is no national registry of such institutions operating in the Philippines.

The documents submitted by the institutions participating in the contests profile the various ways in which they responded to felt needs. These initiatives involved direct provision of health care goods and services, the setting-up of health financing schemes, and activities that simply enhanced or expanded the capacity of the existing health care delivery system (Racelis and Herrin, 1995). Unfortunately, the available data do not indicate the level of health care expenditure by these institutions. Like the HMOs, community-based financing institutions and delivery systems do not fall under any government's regulatory system for the understandable reason that they are hard to identify and monitor.

9.4   RECENT LAWS AND THEIR POTENTIAL EFFECTS ON THE PRIVATE HEALTH SECTOR

Several recent laws are likely to have an impact on the further growth and development of the private health sector *vis-à-vis* the public health sector. However, it is too early to determine the effects of these laws. The brief discussion below will therefore be necessarily speculative. The first set of laws affects the demand for private health care, while the second affects the composition of private health care providers.

9.4.1   The Local Government Code

The first law is the Local Government Code, which devolves the provision and financing of health services to the local government units. Different scenarios are possible. One is that the local governments will mobilize additional local resources to expand the local public sector health delivery system. This could shift the balance between the public and private health sectors, if the private sector does not expand in tandem. On the other hand, the local government units could instead promote the expansion of the local private sector through direct purchases of private sector services or by establishing local insurance and other financing schemes. This would expand private sector provision relative to the government sector.

9.4.2 The National Health Insurance Act

The second important law is the National Health Insurance Act of 1995, which establishes a national health insurance program. This program expands the current Medicare Program to cover the entire population of the country. The National Insurance Program came into effect in 1996.

A key feature of this program is the coverage of indigents, whose premiums will be subsidized by the central and local governments. One could expect an increased demand for health services arising from such coverage. This could provide an added impetus to the growth of the private sector. However, the expected demand — and, therefore, the consequent private health sector impact — would depend on the level of benefits that the insurance program would provide. Limited funding by the government to subsidize the premiums of indigents would mean limited benefits, and limited demand creation, at least by the indigent population. The implementation of the National Insurance Program, however, could lead to a number of organizational innovations in the delivery of health care by the private sector in its attempt to increase its share of the expanded health care market. The development of local HMOs might be a possibility.

9.4.3 Magna Carta of Public Health Workers

A third law, called the Magna Carta of Public Health Workers of 1992, provides for significant increases in salaries and benefits, better working conditions, and security of tenure, among other things. These benefits could raise worker morale and thereby improve the quality of public health services. This might draw consumers away from the private sector and bring back those who went to the private sector because of poor quality of service in the public sector.[7] This could in turn reduce the size of the private health sector, all things being equal.

On the other hand, the provision of all these benefits, especially by the local governments, which will now have to pay for them under the devolution of health services, may raise the cost of providing care, with consequent pressure on local budgets. Local governments might then consider providing services to their constituents at lower cost through direct purchases of cheaper private sector services where available. Alternatively, they could simply consider privatizing some public facilities to reduce the pressure on the public budget.

9.4.4 Philippine Midwifery Act

In addition to these major laws that are likely to have a profound impact on the health system in general, and the role of the private sector in particular, there is

---

[7]Data from the 1987 National Health Survey showed that, among users of various health facilities, about 10 per cent reported dissatisfaction with public hospitals and public primary care facilities, while only 3 per cent or less said they were dissatisfied with private hospitals.

legislation dealing mainly with legally delimiting the task performed by certain professionals. The first is the Philippine Midwifery Act of 1992. Among its provisions is the imposition of penalties on any person practising midwifery in the Philippines without a certificate of registration. To be issued a certificate of registration, however, one has first to graduate from government-recognized and duly accredited institutions and then pass a board examination.

This means that the traditional birth attendants (hilots) would no longer qualify to practise (for pay) their usual trade. The law that this one amended had allowed traditional birth attendants to continue in the practice of their trade provided they were registered with the DOH as having been trained under its program. This provision allowing trained hilots to practise has been deleted from the present law. This law will probably be difficult to enforce given the fact that, as shown earlier, a large proportion of women still rely on traditional birth attendants for their deliveries. If it can be enforced, then the composition of the private sector would change: one category of provider is legally substituted for another. This implies increased costs for consumers.

9.4.5   Revised Optometry Law

Among its provisions, the Revised Optometry Law of 1995 now allows optometrists to use diagnostic drugs. Ophthalmologists, who lobbied against the passage of the law, are generally against optometrists and non-doctors of medicine applying pharmaceutical agents to the human eye. As in the case of the midwives, there is the potential trade-off that is difficult to assess. There is a trade-off between higher quality (purportedly achieved by legally limiting the tasks performed according to the nature of the training obtained) and lower costs for consumers from greater provider substitution.

9.5   CONCLUSION

The private health sector in the Philippines is as large as the public sector, whether one looks at it from the point of view of financing, of health facilities and providers, or of health services utilization. Both sectors grew rapidly in the 1970s, partly due to the stimulus provided by Medicare. The growth of the private sector, however, at least in terms of hospital facilities, slowed down in the 1980s. This slow growth is partly due to the effects of the economic crisis.

In the longer run, the development of the private health sector is influenced by the overall performance of the economy. The slow economic growth and the slow structural transformation in the last two decades have prevented a more rapid growth of the private health sector. On the other hand, government policies have stimulated private sector development by encouraging the production of health providers and special financing for private hospital construction, by mandating employers to provide for health benefits to their employees, and by initiating social insurance. As the private sector has developed, it has been necessary to continually assure high quality of care. Indeed, a number of government regulations were implemented for this purpose. These have included the regulation of health professionals and health care facilities.

Recently, a number of laws have been passed that would have profound impacts on the health sector in general, and the role of the private sector in particular. These include the devolution of health services to local government units, the establishment of a national health insurance program that will provide universal coverage, and a bill of rights for public health workers, providing them with more benefits. In addition, there is legislation that legally limits the tasks performed by certain professionals. To date, however, information on the effects of these laws is not available.

REFERENCES

Griffin, C.C., Alano, B., Ginson-Bautista, M., Gamboa, R.M. (1994). *The Private Medical Sector in the Philippines.* Health Finance Development Project Monograph No. 4. Manila: Health Finance Development Project, Philippines Department of Health, United States Agency for International Development and UPecon Foundation.

Herrin, A., Racelis, R. (1994). Monitoring the coverage of public programs on low-income families in the Philippines, 1992. National Economic and Development Authority. National Statistical Coordination Board (NSCB). *1994 Philippine Statistical Yearbook.* Manila: NSCB.

Herrin, A., Russo, G., Pons, M. (1992). *Priority Health Issues: A Case Study on the Philippines.* Paper prepared for Regional Conference on Priority Health and Population Issues sponsored by the Asian Development Bank and East-West Center Population Institute, Honolulu.

National Statistics Office and Macro International, Inc. (1994a). *Philippines National Demographic Survey 1993.* Calverton, Maryland: National Statistics Office and Macro International, Inc.

National Statistics Office and Macro International, Inc. (1994b). *Philippines National Safe Motherhood Survey 1993.* Calverton, Maryland: National Statistics Office and Macro International, Inc.

Patao, D., Jeffers, J. (1994). *Profile of Medicare Program II Target Beneficiaries.* Health Finance Development Project Monograph No. 8. Manila: Philippines Department of Health, USAID, and Management Sciences for Health.

Racelis, R., Herrin, A. (1994). *National Health Accounts of the Philippines: Partial Estimates as of November 1994.* Paper prepared for the Conference Pesos for Health Part Two: Emerging Results of Current Research on Health Care Reform, sponsored by UPecon Foundation, Health Policy Development Program.

Racelis, R., Herrin, A. (1995). *Community-Based Health Initiatives in the Philippines.* Manila: Health Policy Development Program and UPecon Foundation.

Reyes, E., Picazo, O. (1990). *Health Manpower Employment and Productivity in the Philippines.* Working Paper Series No. 90-19, Philippine Institute for Development Studies.

Rodriguez, A., Briones, R., Teh, R. Jr. (1993). *The Regulatory Environment in the Health Care Sector.* Paper prepared for Philippine Institute for Development Studies.

Solon, O., Gamboa, R., Schwartz, J., Herrin, A. (1991). *Health Sector Financing in the Philippines*, Vol. II. Research Triangle Institute and University of the Philippines School of Economics.

Solon, O., Sumulong, L.R., Tan, C.A. Jr., Capuno, J.J., Quinsing, P.F., Alabastro, S.F. (1995). *The Challenge of Health Care Financing Reforms in the Philippines.* Report presented at the National Workshop on Baseline Research on Health Care Finance, sponsored by Philippines Department of Health and Philippines Institute for Development Studies.

Part IV

Quality of Care Issues and Lessons

10

Quality of Care Issues in Health Sector Reform

WILLIAM NEWBRANDER

Health Economist, Management Sciences for Health

and

GERALD ROSENTHAL

Health Economist, Management Sciences for Health

10.1   INTRODUCTION

Serious resource constraints have led to an overriding concern in most countries to find the means for generating more revenues for health, especially in the public sector. Providers are also concerned about scarce resources. For example, if physicians do not have sufficient supplies, drugs, staff, or facilities due to lack of resources, they cannot maintain professional standards of care. These concerns have led to intensified efforts and policy discussions to find financing mechanisms that will increase available resources for the system, including user fees, cost sharing, or patient contributions.

Some observers believe, however, that such financing mechanisms will not work. Because of the poor quality of services in the public sector, people are unwilling to pay for these services. Unless there are demonstrable quality improvements, demand will remain low and the additional revenues will not be realized. The impact of quality on utilization was shown in a recent UNICEF (1995) Bamako Initiative baseline study of public sector primary health care services. This study found that, in one district in Pakistan, the community saw no value in using local health facilities for necessary care due to the low quality of care there: only 5 per cent of sick children were taken to local health facilities for treatment. Only with adequate levels of quality will patients and purchasers, such as insurers, be willing to pay for services that they formerly received at no or minimal cost. Others claim that quality improvements can be made only after fees are collected and revenues made available for enhancing quality.

A corollary concern, in light of the scarcity of resources, has been the issue of "value for money". If resources are scarce, then the existing ones must be used in the

Private Health Sector Growth in Asia: Issues and Implications. Edited by W. Newbrander.
© 1997 John Wiley & Sons, Ltd.

most effective and efficient manner possible. Neither the government nor other financiers of health services, such as insurers, are willing to provide health services for their clients if the services are of no benefit to the patients. This desire to ensure that the services provided with existing resources provide value for money has led to increased interest in quality of care. Hence, countries are interested not only in augmenting their current resources to increase the quantity of health services but also in the quality of those services.

The objectives of this chapter are to define quality; to examine how it can be measured; to discuss what factors influence quality; to review the methods for improving quality; to evaluate the relationship between quality and costs; to explore any differences in quality between the public and private sectors; and to propose ways in which the public and private sectors can collaborate to promote improvements in the quality of care.

10.2   WHAT IS QUALITY?

10.2.1   Definition of quality

Quality of care is difficult to define. The term is generally considered an evaluative statement (judgment) of the process of care. Although it has been discussed and measured over the years, no single comprehensive definition of quality has evolved. This is because it is multifaceted. Donabedian (1980, 1982, 1985), the most renowned expert on quality, realized its complexity and approached its study in steps. Hence, to come up with a precise and universally agreed-upon definition of quality has proven elusive.[1] However, we may use some of the commonly accepted concepts to guide our discussion.

When the generic term quality of care is used, most people are referring to what we would call the *technical* aspects of quality, such as the provider's behavior and skill in making interventions and applying technology.[2] Donabedian (1980), however, points out that the basic components of care are both the technical quality of care and the management of the interpersonal process. These *interpersonal* elements of quality are judged as good or bad according to how the care complies with social norms, ethical standards, clients' expectations, and amenities. There are also *social* elements of quality that are nonclinical in nature. These nontechnical aspects include accessibility of the services, the efficiency with which they are delivered, and the convenience of using the services.

This structuring of the concept of quality of care assesses the expected interaction between a health provider and the recipient of those services. It involves an evaluation of care on a case-by-case basis. But quality of care also relates more generally to the population and the health system and must be assessed in the general patterns of care and services available to the public.

---

[1]See Chapter 1 of De Geynt (1995) for a detailed review of definitions of quality and its objectives.
[2]Here technical quality of care is maximized when the provider facilitates the optimal balance of expected benefits and risk or expected harm from care.

10.2.2   Dimensions of quality

While there is no agreed-upon definition of quality, some dimensions of quality have emerged from the work done in this field. The dimensions of care are interrelated and, although not all are of equal importance, each has a bearing on quality. For example, Mongkolsmai (see Chapter 6) found evidence of the private sector in Thailand competing with the public sector on the nonclinical aspects of quality, such as use of expensive imported technology, providing convenient locations, being open during evening hours, having much shorter waiting times, and increasing hospital amenities.

Some of the dimensions of quality that are commonly accepted are excellence and appropriateness of the clinical care rendered as judged by professional and societal norms, access, interpersonal relations or patient satisfaction, efficiency, continuity of care, consistency of care, and effectiveness of care. Table 10.1 provides a typology under the broad headings of technical, interpersonal, and social aspects of quality of care. From these elements, it is evident that quality is determined not solely by professional service providers but also by patients and society.

Table 10.1. Dimensions of Quality of Care.

1. Technical aspects of Quality
    Accuracy of diagnosis
    Efficacy of treatment
    Excellence according to professional standards
    Necessity of care
    Appropriateness
    Continuity of care
    Consistency

2. Interpersonal aspects of Quality
    Patient satisfaction
    • Acceptability of care
    • Time spent with provider
    • Attitudes of provider and treatment by staff
    Amenities

3. Social aspects of Quality
    Efficiency
    Accessibility

10.2.3   A framework for assessing quality

If quality is a judgment of care, how can it be assessed? Although there is not a common definition of quality, there has been close to universal agreement on a basic conceptual framework for assessing quality. Donabedian's (1988) framework, which has been accepted and modified by others, uses the elements of structure, process, and outcomes. As he noted, these three elements describe approaches for gathering and analyzing information about quality rather than being the actual attributes of quality. All three elements relate to the provision of care.

Structure describes the attributes of the setting within which care is delivered. It is a static description of the relation of the structure of care to the actual process. This relationship is not well understood and is not directly causal. For instance, the study by Thomason and Edwards (1991) in Papua New Guinea of the structural elements of care at provincial hospitals found that the absence of certain equipment, facilities, management practices, staff, and drugs was likely to result in poor quality but that the presence of those items did not assure high quality.

The outcomes of care are a measure of the patient's present and future health status attributable to the process of care. Outcomes of care make the successful use of care the measure of quality. As Donabedian notes, outcomes must be *relevant* to the goal, *achievable* by good care, and *attributable* to the care evaluated. The measure of outcomes may be immediate, short term, or long term.

Process is the primary concern in attempting to assess quality. It relates to the actual interaction between provider and client or patient. There is a causal link between the outcomes of care and what occurs during the process. Structure and outcomes are actually indirect means for assessing the process of care.

Within these elements, there are three bases upon which judgments of quality are made. These are *criteria,* which are the attributes of structure, process, or outcomes; *norms,* which are general rules of what is good; and *standards,* which are the specific quantitative measures that define goodness.

10.3   WHY IS QUALITY IMPORTANT?

10.3.1   *Improved outcomes*

The basic reason for assessing and upgrading the quality of care is to improve the outcomes of care. Improved outcomes should result in reduced mortality and morbidity. Better-quality care will improve not only the technical but also the interpersonal aspects of care, which are positively related to the outcomes of care. There are a number of other interrelated reasons for measuring and enhancing the quality of care.

10.3.2   *Social interest in quality*

Society has several interests in enhancing quality. First, it has an interest in ensuring that health providers carry out their responsibilities properly and adhere to certain norms and standards. This applies not only to the technical aspects of care but also to providers' interpersonal behavior with patients.

Second, society has an interest in how resources are used. Quality is one determinant of costs and affects the efficiency with which health resources are utilized. As mentioned above, the financiers of care — government, insurers, employers, and consumers — want to know that what they are buying and receiving gives them value for money. With large expenditures for medical care, those who are paying for services want to be assured that the patient is receiving good care. They also want to know whether the care provided was justified.

Third, society is interested in equity. If care is accessible to all but the quality of that care varies widely, there is an equity problem. Studies in many developed and developing countries indicate that access to good-quality care is closely related to a patient's income level, education, social class, and geographic location.

Finally, social interest in the quality of care has been aroused because of new organizational forms, such as health maintenance organizations (HMOs), which have been introduced in health care delivery systems in many countries. While these new forms have some positive effects (such as improved efficiency), they can also have some unintended and undesirable effects (for example, reducing quality expenses by inappropriately reducing the lengths of stay of patients to minimize expenses). While these new organizational forms may achieve certain desirable social objectives, such as efficient resource allocation, they should not do so at the expense of other objectives, such as maintaining or improving quality. For example, outpatient surgical centers in Cali, Colombia, were introduced to save resources. These centers had to prove to the medical establishment, their patients, and the community that the care provided in this alternative setting was not only less costly but also of better quality.

10.3.3 Consumers' interest in quality

The government must assume some of the responsibility for protecting the public from poor-quality care. This role is necessary because health care does not fit the traditional definition of an economic good where consumers have perfect information about the product and can therefore make logical economic choices based on the price and quality of the good. With health care services, there is the need to assist the public in assessing the technical aspects of quality since these are more difficult for patients to assess than the interpersonal aspects of quality. Bhat (see Chapter 8) illustrates some of the dynamics of these legal efforts to protect consumers from poor quality. Recently the recipients of care in many countries — both individually and collectively — have begun to play a more active role in assessing the quality of the care they receive, to ensure that it is of a reasonable standard.

10.3.4 Providers' interest in quality

Providers have an economic interest in providing high-quality care. Improved quality will increase demand for services. This is based on the assumption that quality is important to patients and greatly influences their choice of a health service provider. Thus, private sector providers, who are dependent on generating demand for their services to generate revenues, will have a greater propensity to seek to improve quality than public sector providers, who are not dependent on demand. Since consumers' perceptions of quality are often based on the interpersonal aspects of care, private providers often seek to make improvements in such areas as the surroundings in which care is provided, amenities, and increased use of technology.

Providers also have a professional interest in technical quality, since it provides a means for improving their performance and fulfilling their professional responsibilities. The professional ethic among health professionals dictates that they do what is best in the patient's interests, which usually means providing the best-quality care possible. De Geynt (1995) classifies this as self-regulation or self-correction; there is an educational purpose for measuring and enhancing health care quality.

Thus providers in the public sector may have a professional interest in improving quality but are generally not concerned about improving quality to generate demand for their services. However, this is changing as public sector facilities try to increase demand in order to increase revenues; they too are now attempting to enhance the amenities and surroundings of care.

10.3.5   Consequences and costs of poor quality

Maintaining and improving the quality of care is also important because poor-quality care has individual and social costs associated with it. Poor-quality health care may have undesirable clinical and economic effects. These include costs due to harmful care, ineffective care, and the waste of scarce financial resources. In addition, and possibly more important, consistently poor-quality care in public sector facilities undermines the credibility of the health delivery system with patients and the population in general.

The increased morbidity and mortality resulting from poor quality may result in higher social costs, such as lost productivity, additional health care costs, and increased costs for social insurance. Such costs may be higher than most people suspect. In the USA, it has been estimated that 5 per cent of all hospital admissions are due to nosocomial diseases, which cost billions of dollars to treat (Parker and Newbrander, 1994). In addition to these costs, there was 4 per cent morbidity among these patients. The ability to measure some of these costs is quite limited, but officials must balance the costs of quality improvement against the benefits of having good-quality and effective health services.

On the clinical side, poor quality sometimes results in no change in the patient's condition because the treatment was incomplete or inadequate (for example, the use of poor-quality drugs). Harmful care, on the other hand, can prolong an illness or even cause death. Improper treatment may occur when the provider has not maintained clinical standards, or it can be a result of other factors, such as a breakdown in the drug procurement and supply system.

On the economic side, limited financial resources may be wasted on poor-quality services. Ineffective care, unnecessary care, or harmful care may lead to possible additional care or more costly treatments. When the waste of limited financial resources is multiplied many times, the cumulative effect is a health system that is ineffective in dealing with real health problems.

In addition to adverse clinical and economic effects, poor quality may gravely undermine the credibility of the health system. A number of studies, including a recent one (Newbrander, 1995), show that poor quality in the form of drug shortages may discourage people from using any public facilities. Health workers' morale may also be affected, particularly if drug shortages are so common that it is impossible for them to treat patients properly.

10.4   DOES QUALITY DIFFER BETWEEN THE PUBLIC AND PRIVATE SECTORS?

In many countries, it is assumed that the quality of care in the private sector is higher than that in the public sector. Indicators such as stock-outs of drugs, lack of equipment or broken equipment, poorly maintained facilities, and inadequately trained and supervised health workers are some of the measures used to "prove" quality problems in the public sector health facilities. Are these assessments consistent with available evidence? The number of actual studies of quality is limited. The studies dealing with technical quality are more numerous than those dealing with interpersonal aspects of care.

10.4.1   Technical quality differences

De Geynt reviewed 22 published quality of care studies done in developing countries between 1981 and 1993. All the studies examined technical quality. None of them assessed quality based on outcome indicators: a third used structural indicators to measure quality, over half used process indicators, and the remainder used a combination of structural and process indicators. Few of these compared public and private facilities. Of those that did, mission hospitals and health centers were found to have better quality (Vogel, 1989). None of the studies evaluated the quality of private for-profit providers and facilities.

In a study of rural health facilities in Papua New Guinea (Garner *et al.*, 1990), the private mission health centers were found to have a higher quality of care than the government health centers. The study used structural indicators to assess quality. It reviewed the performance of the health centers in basic but essential tasks, such as immunizations, and in adherence to treatment protocols, as well as assessing their staffing, equipment, and facilities. Two explanations for their ability to offer higher-quality care were that the mission health centers had more staff and used more money to operate. However, lest it be implied that outside factors such as budgets are the sole cause of high or poor quality of care, the authors noted that the mission centers had better communication, supervision, and maintenance.

A cost study of government facilities (Fabricant and Newbrander, 1994) used structural indicators and found that the reference private mission facilities provided higher-quality care based on those indicators. The higher quality was evidenced by fewer drug stock-outs, better-trained and supervised staff, more functional essential equipment, and better maintenance of the equipment and facilities. The demand for health services at the mission facilities was much greater, in part due to their higher quality. These mission facilities drew their patients from a much wider geographical area than the comparable government facilities.

10.4.2   Interpersonal relations and patient satisfaction

The few existing studies of the interpersonal dimensions of care (from the perspective of patient satisfaction) examine quality only tangentially. These studies cite similar reasons why patients are not satisfied with public sector health services:

long waiting times, discourteous staff, providers giving insufficient time and attention to patients' problems, insufficient staff, irregular hours, frequent lack of drugs or other necessary supplies such as X-ray films, crowded wards and clinics, lack of equipment or inoperable equipment, and poorly maintained physical facilities (Berman and Rannan-Eliya, 1993). In Chapter 9 on the Philippines, Herrin cites a study that found that more patients were dissatisfied with public hospitals and primary health care facilities than with private hospitals.

Poor perceptions of quality of care by communities result in decreased demand. Many seek alternative sources of care, such as mission facilities, even if they are much more distant. In other situations, poor-quality care in public facilities has resulted in patients deferring care until the need was acute or life threatening or shifting to self-care, such as purchasing drugs from a kiosk (Newbrander, 1995).

10.4.3   Perceptions of higher quality in the private sector

Most studies examine quality at public or private facilities but not both. There is a paucity of studies comparing public and private facilities and even fewer studies examining quality of private for-profit providers. In addition, most studies are done in rural settings and do not address the issues in the urban settings.

If the existing studies show that mission facilities provide higher-quality care, the next question is why? There are several possible explanations. First, the staff of mission facilities are more homogeneous; they share the same values and motives for being health providers. Their motives are altruistic and this is positively reflected in the provision of better interpersonal quality of care. The staff at these facilities are usually better motivated and have higher morale because of the work conditions. Second, the private sector is less constrained by regulations and bureaucracy and thus is better equipped to be responsive to market changes. Thus they may be more responsive to consumer needs and desires, which, in turn, will positively affect the demand for their services.

Despite the lack of quantitative evidence (except in the case of mission facilities), the common perception that the private sector, especially for-profit elements, provides higher quality remains. This common perception seems to be a result of several factors: much of the available evidence is based on anecdotes about interpersonal aspects rather than systematic evaluation of technical aspects of quality of care; the existing assessments often confuse technical aspects with interpersonal aspects of quality; and the reviewers sometimes mistakenly assume that market indicators, such as demand for services, constitute an implicit vote by consumers about which health services provide the highest quality.

10.5   THE EFFECTS OF FINANCING SYSTEMS AND PROVIDER PAYMENT MECHANISMS ON QUALITY

The financing and supply sides of the market affect the quality of services provided through the incentives created by these systems.

10.5.1 Financing systems

The increased level of health sector reform in many countries of Asia has resulted, in part, from the increased reliance on markets to allocate resources to health. This trend has had an impact on the quality of health care services. For example, in Korea, the extended use of insurance has created tremendous increases in demand for health services as well as demand for increased quality of services among the public (Yang, 1995).

This example illustrates a key principle: the price of health care is a major determinant of demand for health care, the consumer's choice of provider, and the level of quality of care. If countries are using markets for allocation decisions, then this choice will provide incentives for private providers to increase quality, possibly in its interpersonal and amenities aspects rather than its technical elements. Hence in a truly market-driven health setting, private providers will have the incentive to increase quality, even if it is not technical quality, to attract additional patients. This was the case in Thailand, where hospitals stress their quality differences in marketing.

The willingness of users of health services to pay for quality has been studied. In general, it has been found that quality of care is important in determining users' demand and utilization patterns for health care providers. Such findings are based on many indirect measures of these demand factors for quality. For example, Denton *et al.* (1991) examined the question of how quality changes would affect demand for health services. They found that improvements in quality would significantly increase demand for services. Patients were willing to pay for these quality increases. Improvements would have a larger impact on increasing demand than lower prices. However, these findings were not observed changes but were simulations from the data.

Wouters (1991) reviewed a number of the studies of willingness to pay for health services. Some of these studies used crude assessment instruments to determine quality levels, implying that consumers' willingness to pay indirectly reflects quality. The demand studies reviewed by Wouters suggested that quality was an important decision variable for users choosing a provider and that they were willing to pay for quality improvements. Since these studies relied on structural assessments of quality, they found that the most important variable was the availability of drugs. There was a much weaker relationship between choice of provider and other aspects of quality, such as amenities, properly maintained facilities, and type of provider. Though these studies provide some information, many questions remain: How sensitive is demand to quality changes? Do such findings apply equally to public and private sector health facilities? Do problems with drug supplies overemphasize preferences for availability of drugs as a key element of quality?

Other payers of services (government and insurers) may promote better quality by monitoring the services purchased for their clients. As indicated above, introduction of new organizational forms, such as HMOs, that combine the functions of the financing and provision of health services, must be closely monitored to ensure that quality is maintained.

10.5.2   Provider payment mechanisms

The payment system has a direct effect on the incentives or disincentives created for providing high-quality care. This makes it imperative that the effects of payment systems on quality be considered before their introduction. The perceived difference in quality between public and private facilities may help support the presence and growth of the private sector. The public sector may have more health facilities and bed capacity in some areas yet the private sector may continue to grow in these areas due to perceived differences in quality by health users. The differences of quality between the private and public sectors may be negative or positive. Private providers face incentives to increase quality while simultaneously facing other incentives to decrease quality. For instance, private providers may have the incentive to increase quality in order to influence the choice users will make among alternative providers. They may purchase equipment and have the necessary supplies and drugs for proper treatment of patients so that there is increased demand for their services. It has also been noted that private providers have greater incentives, freedom, and ability to provide higher-quality services than public providers with respect to the nontechnical aspects of quality (Berman and Rannan-Eliya, 1993).

However, quality may be decreased if a payment system is based on the number of services provided. Providers may order more tests, provide more services or extend hospital length of stay longer than necessary. Unnecessary care, even if not harmful, represents a lower level of quality. This has happened in Korea with the proliferation of technology and expansion of providers and their services (see Chapter 5 by Yang).

Table 10.1 illustrates the means by which payment methods may influence the behavior of providers and patients — and ultimately quality. It reviews various payment systems for hospitals, their expected responses, effects on patients, and potential effects on quality. It shows the multiple and complicated ways in which payment mechanisms may create positive or negative incentives.

10.6   OPERATIONAL METHODS FOR ENSURING AND IMPROVING QUALITY

While many developed countries have directed their attention to monitoring and evaluating the quality of health services, developing countries have been dealing with the critical issues of adequate resources and access. Because their focus has been on maintaining existing health service levels while expanding population coverage, the issue of the quality of services has arisen more recently for these countries.

The question is how to improve quality. A number of methodologies have been developed to deal with improving the quality of services. Some of these methodologies or models have been developed specifically for the health care setting, while others have taken a generic model from the business world and sought to apply its principles to health. These models include quality assurance (QA), quality improvement, continuous quality improvement, and total quality management (TQM).

There are various ways to improve the technical and interpersonal aspects of quality, but all the methodologies usually have four basic elements in common:

Table 10.2. Incentives for Hospitals under Various Payment Methods and their Impact on Patients and Quality.

Method of reimbursement	Hospital incentive	Impact on patient	Positive quality impact if:	Negative quality impact if:
Charges				
Full	Increase charges	Increase utilization	Cost concerns limit services to essential services	Cost concerns result in insufficient services
Percentage	Increase charges	Increase utilization but with restraint	Cost concerns limit services to essential services	Cost concerns result in insufficient services
Fixed fee	Increase costs more slowly	Uncertain	Cost concerns limit services to essential services	Cost concerns prevent provision of essential services
Costs				
Retrospective	Increase charges and costs	Increase utilization	More services that are needed are used	Services are over-used or unnecessary
Prospective	Increase charges and costs more slowly	Increase utilization	Provider offers more services than required	Too many services are used
Formulas				
Per day	Increase LOS	Later discharge	Longer stay appropriate for condition	LOS is too long for condition
Per admission	Increase admissions, decrease LOS	Earlier discharge	Case is uncomplicated	Patient is admitted too often or discharged too soon
Per diagnosis	Increase admissions, more complex case mix, decrease LOS	Earlier discharge	Case is uncomplicated	Case is difficult
Fixed Annual Budget	Limit admissions, decrease LOS	Earlier discharge	Care is appropriate	Skimping on care with shorter LOS
Capitation	Limit admissions, decrease LOS	Earlier discharge	Shorter stay is technically appropriate	Skimping on LOS when longer stay is medically appropriate

LOS, Length of stay.

(1) setting standards, (2) disseminating those standards, (3) identifying problems of compliance with the standards through monitoring the process, and (4) correcting problems and improving the process. All these methodologies are based on the premise that to improve quality, the process by which care is provided must be improved.

This chapter is not intended to provide a comprehensive review of the various models for improving quality, since there are other sources that do this. This section briefly presents some of the characteristics of these models for assuring and improving quality. Gani's discussion in Chapter 11 of the Unit Swadana hospitals in Indonesia illustrates the practical application of quality assurance and quality management to a specific health care setting. There are other simple, low-cost methods that may prove useful for assessing quality.[3]

10.6.1   Elements of quality assurance and improvement

QA is the oldest and most familiar form of quality improvement. It involves assessing care that has already been provided and taking action to improve it in the future. This is done by identifying problems in health service delivery, analyzing those problems, and seeking to solve them. This analysis is based on the two elements Donabedian (1980, 1982, 1985) identified: technical care and the management of the interpersonal process between the provider and the patient.

The process of improving quality is more complicated; it requires further definition of the components of QA. The USAID Quality Assurance Project has identified a 10-step process for QA:[4]

1. Planning for quality assurance
2. Developing guidelines and setting standards
3. Communicating standards and specifications
4. Monitoring quality
5. Identifying problems and selecting opportunities for improvement
6. Defining the problem operationally
7. Choosing a team
8. Analyzing and studying the problem to identify its root causes
9. Developing solutions and actions for improvement
10. Implementing and evaluating quality improvement efforts.

The focus of most QA work is a hospital or clinic setting. The work of the Quality Assurance Project in many developing countries has expanded the scope of QA activities to include primary health care and family planning services.

---

[3]See, for example, Thomason and Edwards (1991).
[4]University Research Corporation, Chevy Chase, MD.

10.6.2   Methodologies

Although there are several different methods of QA, an overriding concern of many QA programs is that of health care costs. As mentioned above, insurers want to know if their beneficiaries are receiving necessary and good-quality care.

10.6.2.1 Information for assessing quality. Any quality assessment requires information about the process of care in order to compare it with a standard of what should occur. Studies have focused on various kinds of facilities: outreach services, physicians' offices, and hospital polyclinics and inpatient units. Assessments of primary health care facilities, clinics, and physicians' offices often use structural quality assessments, such as reviewing the equipment available at the facility, the training and qualifications of the staff, and the level of supervision or in-service education provided.

Quality assessments of facilities may also examine process factors, such as undesirable outcomes and preventable deaths. Another concern, especially for an insurer, is care that is not justified. In some countries the percentage of inappropriate admissions is directly related to the type of hospital (for-profit or not-for-profit) and whether the provider is in the public or private sector.

10.6.2.2 Ensuring good quality through structure. The structural method of QA suggests that good quality should be an inherent feature of the system. It means that we should take features that we know lead to appropriate care and build a system with those attributes. For example, we might want to plan a health system or use facilities having the following characteristics: proper financial incentives, good access, appropriate staffing, appropriate range of services and benefits, and proper quality surveillance mechanisms. It is assumed that this system will then provide a high level of quality of care as long as its structural features are monitored and maintained.

10.6.2.3 Ensuring quality through monitoring. Another QA method is to actually perform surveillance or monitor quality. This most frequently happens where there is a basis for licensure, certification, or accreditation of providers. It guarantees that the system is set up according to the proper standards. For instance, licensure — the oldest and most fundamental QA mechanism — is designed to assure the patient that a physician or nurse has a specified level of training relevant to his or her profession and may also require some form of continuing education. This has not proved to be a strong basis for assuring quality.

Voluntary professional certification and accreditation are other pervasive structural QA mechanisms. For physicians, certification by a specialty board may require certain training and special examination. Certification is similar to but goes beyond licensure by setting minimal standards of quality for providers' training and knowledge. For institutions, there may be voluntary accreditation that assesses the organizational structure, qualifications of physicians and nursing staff, and physical environment.

10.6.3 Licensing and regulation

Improving quality through licensing and regulation is a government responsibility. The reasons for government involvement in quality may be a proactive interest in protecting the public. In other instances, it may be self-interest: the government may be a large purchaser of health services and may wish to ensure that what it is purchasing is of an adequate standard.

Licensing is one of the simpler forms of assuring quality through regulation. However, its ability to maintain consistent quality standards is dubious at best because of lax enforcement and the tendency for minimal standards.

Using other regulatory mechanisms to ensure quality can be difficult for countries, since expert judgments are required to assess quality. To be successful, a strong administrative organization must be established and maintained and legal mechanisms for enforcement must be in place. Licensing and regulation are the easiest forms of quality improvement to maintain because they deal with structural aspects of quality and very little with the process or outcome aspects of assessing quality.

10.7   BARRIERS TO IMPROVING QUALITY

Improvement of quality is not necessarily a priority in a health system for a number of reasons including:

- Lack of resources
- Inability of the public and private sectors to work together
- Inadequate information systems
- Lack of organizational structures to promote quality
- Lack of commitment.

Lack of resources is one of the primary reasons some countries give for the lack of initiatives to improve quality of care. A former Secretary of Health for the Philippines asked rhetorically how the Department of Health could be expected to regulate health facilities if only 1 per cent of its resources are dedicated to that effort (Galvez-Tan, 1996). The assumption is that to improve quality requires more resources. This issue will be examined below in the section on costs but suffice it to say that, at times, providing fewer services and goods may lead to higher quality. For instance, better drug prescribing may lead to fewer drugs being provided to patients, at a lower cost and with an improvement in quality of care.

There may be the will to improve quality but inadequate information systems or the organizational structures to do so. Quality assessment and improvement require a tremendous amount of data to establish a baseline for an ongoing monitoring system. The lack of adequate information systems may impede the introduction of QA systems.

Finally, there may be a lack of commitment on the part of the public sector officials (or bodies representing private sector practitioners and institutions) to improve quality. This may be a consequence of lack of information, resources, or resolution to meet the challenge. Or the other preconditions (such as organizational structures, information systems, or regulatory requirements) may not exist.

The key lesson for improving quality is that it must be done throughout the health system and not simply in the public or private sector side. For its part, the public sector may view its role as the "enforcer" over the private sector without any attempt at self-regulation. Such attempts lead to conflict between the public and private sectors and prevent a unified strategy for promotion of quality. The two sectors must work as partners if quality improvement in the health system as a whole is to be a reality.

10.8 QUALITY AND COSTS

Costs are a common concern of all health systems. The escalation of costs of health systems, particularly for the public sector, may be attributed to a number of factors: population growth, demographic and epidemiological changes, an aging population, and new technology.

It is commonly assumed that higher quality means higher costs. The quality improvement methodology assumes that poor quality means higher costs. Is this in fact the case?

10.8.1 How does quality relate to costs?

The findings from a number of studies are inconclusive about a direct relationship between costs and quality. Of the existing studies, it has not been possible to isolate those costs that are directly attributable to quality changes. Often what is termed as a quality improvement is simply ensuring what is necessary to provide basic services.

The relationship between quality and costs has two components, based on the premise that quantity is a necessary precondition for quality. First, there is a relationship between quality and quantity when the quantity of health services is inadequate. Costs may be lower but quality is also lower because of the inadequate quantity of services. If there is an insufficient quantity of health services, the maximum benefit may not be achieved for the patient. Hence, in the short run, costs may have been reduced by minimizing quantity; in the long run, the need for additional care or greater quantity of services may actually cause total costs to be greater than necessary if the correct quantity had been utilized initially.

Second, too much care may mean higher costs and lower quality in two possible ways. Excessive care may increase the probability of harm to the patient. Even if there is not an increased risk of harm, the excessive quantity of services delivered may be considered lower quality because of redundancy and waste of resources. Redundancy is economically inefficient. For example, if more resources are allocated for care than are needed, then there may be fewer resources remaining for other needs.

The basic implications of this relationship of quantity to quality and quantity to cost are: quality costs money; and efficiency gains through reducing unnecessary care may result in the same level of quality but at a lower cost or a higher level of quality for the same cost.

Thus the answer to the question "Does higher quality mean higher costs?" is "not necessarily". In those countries that have faced severe resource constraints, there will be costs associated with bringing standards of practice up to acceptable levels. In this sense, higher quality does mean higher costs. In the Dominican Republic, for example, the resources required to enable the system to reach an acceptable technical standard of quality were estimated to be an additional 30 per cent. However, the provision of higher quality must consider not only the additional costs for inputs to provide a higher standard but should also consider the benefits or cost savings resulting from averting poor quality.

A study of improvements through TQM at the University of Michigan Medical Center found that the value of the quality improvements, after subtracting the costs of TQM, were substantial, amounting to over 3 per cent of the medical center's entire budget. So effective monitoring of quality may actually contain or reduce health care cost increases when this quality improvement results in a significant reduction of unnecessary care and improved clinical treatment procedures.

10.8.2   *How can quality be assured when resources are reduced?*

Some ministries of health assume that reduced resources mean that quality must be decreased. This is certainly the case when an optimal quantity and allocation or type of care delivered must be decreased. Then there can be no increase in the benefits received even if the quantity of services is increased. However, when the mix and quantity of services provided to the population or a specific individual are not optimal, there is room for efficiency gains that may help increase quality without increasing costs.

When resources are constrained or reduced, quality may be increased by examining the allocation of resources to optimize how resources are used to the greatest benefit. Improved technical and economic efficiency may permit increased quality with no increase in resources. For example, if more costly labor inputs are used than necessary to produce the desired service, efficiency can be increased by substituting less costly labor with no change in quality, assuming the labor inputs are equivalent technically.

10.9   HOW CAN THE PUBLIC AND PRIVATE SECTORS IMPROVE QUALITY COLLABORATIVELY?

The public and private sectors can collaborate to improve quality by supporting innovation, improving information for quality monitoring, enhancing clinical and administrative management capacities, and reviewing national programs and project support. Such collaboration is possible because it is straightforward and less controversial than some other areas. However, it may require new approaches to sharing information and experiences and learning about various options, within countries and between countries.

10.9.1   Supporting innovation

The private sector can often be used as a testing ground for new ideas and concepts, including innovative means for assessing and improving quality. Countries may seek the assistance of international agencies in providing resources and encouragement for such experimentation in the private sector which, after it is proved, may be adopted by the public sector. Such an approach may in fact be an indirect means of overcoming resistance to various structural or management changes in those health systems where the public sector predominates.

10.9.2   Improving information for quality monitoring

A major concern of many countries interested in improving quality is the limited information base on quality available to either the public or private sector. There is a need to have information about hospitals, pharmacies, facilities, and providers not only from regular management information systems but also from studies on specific issues of quality. For example:

- It is important to understand the relative cost effectiveness of services offered by public and private sources to understand the relation of costs to quality
- The differences between the public sector's and the private sector's technical quality must be identified and understood if progress is to be made in formulating the proper incentives for providers and financing mechanisms for health services
- Improved information and monitoring systems about public and private health provision and providers' performance will increase knowledge of the quality of existing health services. This would permit improved analysis and monitoring of quality
- Better understanding of health care markets is also needed to understand how the demand and supply factors affect quality and its role in the choices consumers make about certain health services and providers.

10.9.3   Enhancing clinical and administrative management capacities

The complexities of public/private sector interrelationships require the broadest of managerial skills so appropriate planning, implementation, monitoring, and evaluation of quality changes can occur. The skills needed to deal with quality issues are clinical as well as managerial. These will increasingly encompass aspects of regulation of quality and negotiation as the role of the private sector in health grows in relation to that of the public sector. There are many opportunities to strengthen the management capabilities of countries that are seeking closer collaboration between the public and private sectors.

10.9.4   Review of national programs and project support

Allocative efficiency has an influence on quality. Governments and the private sector can examine health funding priorities and budgets to review what is being promoted by such activities. Research is also needed to document and analyze experiences with improving quality so other countries can learn from these lessons.

These recommendations are based on the awareness that major changes are needed in the quality of public and private health services in many countries. In order to make these changes, countries must share experiences, test different models, positively facilitate change to bring about improved quality, and continually monitor the health system — public and private — to ensure that it meets their objectives. International agencies have a role in this process, for example, supplying technical assistance and financial aid, supporting policy reviews, and organizing forums for sharing and disseminating information and experiences among countries grappling with these quality issues related to the public/private mix of services.

10.10   CONCLUSION

Several basic and common assumptions have emerged from this discussion: quality is important to patients and greatly influences their choice of a health service provider, the cost of providing health services is related to the quality of those services, and quality of care is ultimately important because it is necessary for sustaining the health system. Without adequate quality, users will turn to other alternatives. For the public sector, a basic level of quality is necessary if there is to be sufficient demand for its services. Without sufficient demand there will be excess capacity and the credibility of the public health system will be questioned. Private providers of health care face both positive and negative incentives for delivering both high technical quality and high interpersonal quality of services.

It is the challenge of the future to find mechanisms to ensure quality in the public and private sectors. Such efforts require that the public and private sectors find ways to collaborate rather than assuming competitive roles and automatically assigning positions of the "master" and "servant" when seeking compliance with basic quality standards. By working together, they can find innovative, flexible, and system-specific solutions to respond to the unique characteristics of a particular health system. Other countries may observe and learn from such experiences and develop their unique means for improving quality of care.

REFERENCES

Berman, P., Rannan-Eliya, R. (1993). *Factors Affecting the Development of Private Health Care Provision in Developing Countries*. Major Applied Research Paper No. 9. Bethesda, MD: Health Financing and Sustainability Project.

De Geynt, W. (1995). *Managing the Quality of Health Care in Developing Countries*. World Bank Technical Paper No. 258. Washington, DC: World Bank.

Denton, H., Akin, J., Vogel, R., Wouters, A. (1991). *Nigeria: Health Care Costs, Financing and Utilization*. World Bank Sub-Sector Report No. 8382-UNI. Washington, DC: World Bank.

Donabedian, A. (1980). *Explorations in Quality: Assessment and Monitoring, Volume I: The Definition of Quality and Approaches to its Assessment*. Ann Arbor, MI: Health Administration Press.

Donabedian, A. (1982). *Explorations in Quality: Assessment and Monitoring, Volume II: The Criteria and Standards of Quality*. Ann Arbor, MI: Health Administration Press.

Donabedian, A. (1985). *Explorations in Quality: Assessment and Monitoring, Volume III: The Methods and Findings of Quality Assessment and Monitoring: An Illustrated Analysis*. Ann Arbor, MI: Health Administration Press.

Donabedian, A. (1988). The quality of care: how can it be assessed? *JAMA*, **260**(12), 1743–1748.

Fabricant, S., Newbrander, W. (1994). *The Gambia: Health Facilities Cost Study*. Report prepared for the Government of Gambia and the World Bank. Boston: Management Sciences for Health.

Galvez-Tan, J. (1996). *Love, Courtship and Marriage, Health Care Style: Challenges to Partnerships of the Public and Private Sector in Health Care*. Keynote Address, Second Regional Conference on Health Sector Reform: Issues Related to Private Sector Growth. Asian Development Bank, 5–7 March 1996, Manila.

Garner, P., Thomason, J., Donaldson, D. (1990). Quality assessment of health facilities in rural Papua New Guinea. *Health Policy and Planning*, **5**(1): 49–59.

Newbrander, W. (1995). *Equity and Coverage of Health Care Provision in Kenya*. Report prepared for the BASICS Project. Arlington, VA: Partnership for Child Health Care.

Parker, D., Newbrander, W. (1994). Tackling wastage and inefficiency in the health sector. *World Health Forum*, **15**(2), 107–113.

Thomason, J., Edwards, K. (1991). Using indicators to assess quality of hospital services in Papua New Guinea. *Int J Hlth Planning and Management*, **6**, 309–324.

UNICEF. (1995). *The State of the Public Sector Primary Health Care Services District Sheikhupura, Punjab, Pakistan*. Bamako Initiative Technical Report Series No. 31.

Vogel, R. (1989). *Trends in Health Expenditures and Revenue Sources in Sub-Saharan Africa*. Paper prepared for World Bank Sub-Saharan Africa Health Policy Study.

Wouters, A. (1991). Essential national health research in developing countries: health-care financing and the quality of care. *Int J Hlth Planning and Management*, **6**(4), 253–271.

Yang, B. (1995). *Health Care System of Korea: What Now and What in the Future?* Paper presented at the Asian Development Bank First Regional Conference on Health Sector Reform in Asia, 22–25 May 1995, Manila.

11

Improving Quality in Public Sector Hospitals in Indonesia

ASCOBAT GANI

Dean, School of Public Health, University of Indonesia

11.1 INTRODUCTION

Indonesia experienced a remarkably rapid and successful expansion of its health services during the 1970s. At that time, significant revenues were secured from oil exports, which enabled the government to spend more on social welfare. However, declining oil prices from the mid-1970s to the early 1980s taxed the government's available resources, including its health sector budget. A World Bank study (1987) revealed that government hospitals were suffering from insufficient funds; only 40 per cent of the actual operational and maintenance budget was being met. Health centers, which offer 18 basic programs related to primary health care, were similarly short of funds.

Limited resources constrained the government's ability to respond adequately to growing demands for high-quality health services. These demands resulted from demographic and epidemiological changes and rapid socioeconomic development during the previous 25 years (Jeffers, 1990). At present, Indonesia has a population of 195 million with a growth rate of 1.6 per cent annually. Per capita income increased from $600 in 1985 to $919 in 1994. From an epidemiological perspective, there has been a significant increase in chronic degenerative diseases. Cardiovascular diseases have become the number one cause of death, despite the fact that there is still the "unfinished agenda" of combating infectious diseases. Socioeconomic development has created a segment of the population that has the ability to pay for high-quality services. These increased needs and the increased demand for services have created a financing burden for the health sector in Indonesia.

In response to this situation, specific health sector reforms were undertaken. The reforms began 10 years ago and have intensified in the 1990s. The health sector reforms are in the areas of human resources, the pharmaceutical industry, resource mobilization and financing, promotion of the private hospital sector, decentralization, and community and family empowerment through community

Private Health Sector Growth in Asia: Issues and Implications. Edited by W. Newbrander.
© 1997 John Wiley & Sons, Ltd.

financing schemes. One major goal of these reforms has been to mobilize private resources to achieve a more equitable distribution, as well as a higher quality of health services (Bureau of Planning, 1995).

The purpose of this chapter is to present a specific policy initiative in Indonesia that promotes increased autonomy for public hospitals so that they can operate independently, much like private health service providers. This policy, known as "Rumah Sakit Unit Swadana" (RS Unit Swadana), literally means "financially self-sustaining hospital". Since this initiative must be viewed within the context of the current situation in Indonesia, the growth of the private health sector and the various health sector reforms will be described first.

11.1.1   Current situation

During the last 25 years, there has been substantial development within Indonesia's health care infrastructure. This includes the establishment by the government of 5976 health centers, 15 944 health subcenters, and 4024 mobile health centers, to meet the growing need of rural populations for primary health services.

Despite the relatively large infrastructure, national health expenditure in Indonesia remains relatively low as compared to that of its neighbors in Southeast Asia. During the period from 1982 to 1989, national health expenditure amounted to about 2.5 per cent of gross domestic product (GDP) (US $12 per capita annually). Of this amount, the government provided only 30 per cent (about $3 per capita annually). The remaining 70 per cent (or $9) comes from individuals, households, and private firms (Gani, 1990).

This meager public expenditure for the health sector has led to insufficient funds for the operation and maintenance of health services, as well as resulting in lower-quality service in many government hospitals (Bureau of Planning, 1995). In 1990 the government introduced a new policy to limit their number (currently 608 public hospitals), at least until the year 2000.

Insufficient allocations in the government budget, especially for hospitals and health centers, have led to the growth of the private health sector to fill the gap.

11.2   PRIVATE SECTOR PROVISION OF HEALTH CARE

As in other developing countries, the private health sector in Indonesia includes nonprofit and religious organizations, as well as individuals who are licensed (such as private practitioners) or unlicensed practitioners (such as traditional healers). There is a wide range of private sector activities in health care, including providing services, financing, training health providers, and producing and dispensing pharmaceuticals.

The distinction between the public and private sectors is complex with regard to health personnel in Indonesia. This is because most government health personnel, especially doctors and paramedics, also work as private providers, theoretically after office hours. Almost all government doctors who work in health centers also provide outpatient services in their private clinics during the afternoon and evening hours. Similarly, many specialist doctors employed in public hospitals also work in private hospitals or group practice clinics, or have their own private clinics. Although they are allowed to work only after office hours, it is very common for doctors to make visits to private hospitals during government office hours.

Distinctions between the public and private health sectors are also blurred when it comes to the level of services (primary, secondary, and tertiary care), since each level usually provides a mix of services. For example, specialists in solo practice may perform the same treatments as general practitioners (GPs). Similarly, referral hospitals may offer general ambulatory care, which is also provided by health centers.

This chapter will describe two areas of the private provision of health care in Indonesia: (1) the types and characteristics of its primary, secondary, and tertiary care (personnel and facilities); and, (2) utilization patterns. It will differentiate between solo practitioners, outpatient clinics, and hospitals. However, these categories overlap and create statistical problems in defining the private sector due to double counting.

11.2.1 Personnel

Solo practitioners include GPs, specialists, paramedics, midwives, and traditional birth attendants (TBAs). At this time, only doctors and midwives are required to have their clinics registered with the local district and provincial health offices.

11.2.1.1 General practitioners. In 1992, there were 20 276 medical doctors in Indonesia; 14 761 of them were GPs (medical school graduates). In addition, there were 4079 dentists. Since 1975, all medical graduates have been required to serve in government health centers for a period of 2 to 5 years (that is, a graduated scale from 2 years of service in the most remote health centers to 5 years of service in more accessible health centers, such as on Java). In 1992, 6357 medical doctors worked in health centers.

The government adopted a zero growth policy for physicians and stopped recruiting medical doctors in 1992. According to this new policy, new doctors must serve at a government health center for 3 years. Upon completion of their contract, they have three choices: to apply for a government post; to shift to the private sector; or to go for a specialist education. At the beginning of 1995, this first group of contract doctors (1029) finished their contractual services. However, the options for government posting and specialist training opportunities were limited. Without any incentive mechanisms in the rural areas, they are likely to respond to market demand and provide private services in urban areas. One possible mechanism would be to develop community health financing schemes to sustain their staying in subdistrict areas or to support continuing education in the field of family medicine.

As mentioned earlier, almost all doctors have their own clinics. They render outpatient services and, in places where no dispensary is available, they also provide drugs. Doctors in private practice serve around 5 to 50 patients per evening session. Their charges also vary, ranging from Rp 5000 to Rp 15 000, depending on the location and whether or not drugs are included.

It is widely perceived that the quality of service in doctors' private clinics is better than that provided in health centers during office hours. Moreover, doctors are not always available in the health center clinics since they have to perform other functions, including administration and field supervision. It is not clear whether the coexistence of these clinics is competitive or complementary. From a demand point of view, doctors' private clinics offer more choices for those who have the ability to pay for better services.

11.2.1.2 Specialists.   Most of the specialists in Indonesia (5515 in 1992) work in urban areas. Many of these, 28.7 per cent, work in Jakarta, where there is a great demand for specialists' services. Many specialists also provide outpatient services in private clinics outside of office hours. It is not uncommon for specialists to offer services for general health problems, which theoretically could be managed by a GP. In some places this has led to an atmosphere of competition between GPs and specialists.

11.2.1.3 Nurses and paramedics.   In 1992 there was a total of 411975 nurses in Indonesia. A quarter of them were working in hospitals. The rest worked in health centers or as administrators in government health offices. Paramedics, especially those who work in health centers, also provide outpatient services.

11.2.1.4 Midwives.   The midwife (*bidan*) is a traditional private provider of maternity care. Midwives provide antenatal, delivery, and postnatal services. Prior to 1991, their availability in rural areas was limited. The government's commitment to child survival programs has led to a policy of placing a midwife in every village. As of 1991, there were 68 876 villages throughout the country. Of those, 54 116 were in need of a midwife. To meet this need, a special 1-year training course was designed for auxiliary nurses to become village midwives.

The first group of village midwives, numbering 11 883, was placed in 1992. By 1995, the number had increased to 35 000. Village midwives are under contracts similar to those of doctors for 3 years. After the contract period, they are expected to remain in the village and provide maternity care. A survey of several subdistricts in West Java revealed that 75 to 85 per cent of the antenatal care in villages was performed by these midwives. However, when it came to delivery, 95 per cent of pregnant women were assisted by TBAs. The limited number of deliveries assisted by village midwives raises the question as to whether they can afford to stay in the village without sufficient earning capacity. Many will be forced by economic constraints to move to subdistrict capitals or even to the district capital.

11.2.1.5 Traditional birth attendants.   In the 1970s, as part of a policy to provide accessible health care to rural people, the government decided to train TBAs for all villages. They were given training in antenatal and delivery care. Moreover, they were trained to be able to identify difficult cases to be referred to health centers or midwives. Upon completion of their training, the TBAs were equipped with TBA kits (a set of instruments and basic supplies). In practice, TBAs provide comprehensive services, including in-home delivery, cooking, cleaning, and baby care. This makes TBAs more sought after than village midwives. Their payments vary and, in some places, they are paid in kind.

Despite a massive effort to train TBAs, a special study on the quality of their services revealed that there is no significant difference in outcomes of care provided by trained and untrained TBAs.

11.2.2 Facilities

11.2.2.1 Outpatient clinics. Private outpatient clinics are institutionalized facilities in which doctors (GPs or specialists or both) and nurses work in a team to provide ambulatory service. These clinics have an administrative staff and often clinical laboratories. A growing number of these clinics involve group practice by different specialists.

Many of these private outpatient clinics operate in urban and suburban areas, especially in new residential areas in Java, Bali, and Sumatra. Since most of the doctors working in these clinics are government personnel, the clinics may be open in the morning but the doctor is only available in the afternoon and evening.

11.2.2.2 Private hospitals. There were 1039 hospitals in Indonesia in 1994 with a total bed number of 116 847, or one bed for every 1583 population. As demonstrated in Table 11.1, 42 per cent of the hospitals were operated by the private sector, with a total of 37 435 beds (32 per cent).

As mentioned earlier, the government adopted a policy in 1990 to limit the construction of new public hospitals — especially specialist hospitals — at least until the year 2000. The rationale behind this policy was to reduce the government's burden in financing secondary and tertiary care and to allow more funds to be allocated to primary care (Akin *et al.*, 1987). Moreover, studies of several public hospitals revealed that the users of hospital services, which are highly subsidized, came mostly from the higher socioeconomic segments of the population.

Table 11.1. Total Hospitals and Beds, Public and Private, 1989–94.

	1989	1990	1991	1992	1993	1994
Public						
No. of hospitals	599	598	598	602	606	608
% of hospitals	65%	63%	61%	61%	60%	58%
No. of beds	77 896	78 306	78 097	78 607	78 925	79 412
% of beds	73%	72%	70%	70%	69%	68%
Private						
No. of hospitals	325	352	384	392	420	431
% of hospitals	35%	37%	39%	39%	41%	42%
No. of beds	29 216	31 081	33 063	34 172	35 612	37 435
% of beds	27%	28%	30%	30%	31%	32%
Total						
No. of hospitals	924	950	982	994	1026	1039
No. of beds	107 112	109 387	111 160	112 779	114 537	116 847

Source: Data Center of Directorate General of Health Services, Department of Health, Indonesia, 1995.

Although many wealthy Indonesians prefer to be treated abroad, especially for cardiovascular diseases, demand for hospital services in Indonesia has increased. From 1989 to 1994, there was rapid growth in the number of private hospitals. In 1993, for example, 32 new hospitals were constructed: four were public hospitals and the remaining 28 were private hospitals. The proportion of private general hospitals was 27.6 per cent in 1989 but increased to 32.4 per cent by 1994. For specialist hospitals (such as mental, maternity, and ophthalmology), the increase was from 25.3 per cent in 1989 to 30.1 per cent in 1994.

Most of the new private hospitals were constructed in urban areas and many of them in new suburban metropolitan areas (Jakarta, Surabaya, Medan, and Semarang, for example). These new private hospitals are modern, highly specialized, and equipped with sophisticated technology. Most of the private hospitals are owned by domestic investors, usually operating under a nonprofit foundation. However, foreign investors have also begun to enter the hospital industry in Indonesia.

The supply of specialist doctors and qualified hospital nurses has not kept up with the growth in private hospitals. This has created problems for both private and public hospitals. In the past, the government was lenient in allowing its doctors to serve in private hospitals, even during office hours. Now, however, as part of a government policy to improve quality of care in the public hospitals, the Ministry of Health (MOH) in mid-1995 urged private hospitals to recruit their own full-time specialists. Many highly qualified nurses have moved to private hospitals during the last 5 years, partly because of the higher salaries.

11.3   UTILIZATION OF PRIVATE HEALTH CARE

Utilization data are taken from the 1990 National Socio-economic Survey (Susenas). Susenas is a regular national survey undertaken every 3 years. Included in the survey are questions on morbidity and health-seeking behavior (health service utilization) as well as on health expenditure, with a recall period of 1 month. For hospitalization, the recall period is 1 year.

An analysis of the utilization data revealed that private health care providers have been playing a substantial role, mainly in the provision of ambulatory care and maternity care. Preventive services and inpatient care are still dominated by government health services. Utilization of five types of health services — preventive services, ambulatory care, prenatal care, delivery care, and inpatient care — are described below.

11.3.1   Preventive services

The Indonesian population still relies on government facilities for preventive services, specifically immunization. This is apparent from data on immunization coverage reported by government health facilities. In 1991–92, for example, coverage for BCG, DPT, polio, and measles immunization was 95.3, 98.9, 91.3, and 88.6 per cent, respectively.

Table 11.2. Utilization of Public and Private Services by Location and Income Level for Different Services.

		Public	Private	Other[a]
Ambulatory care				
Location	Urban	29.3%	37.2%	33.5%
	Rural	36.4%	31.0%	32.6%
Monthly income (Rp)	> 150 000	30.0%	39.8%	30.2%
	< 150 000	35.6%	30.1%	34.3%
Delivery services				
Location	Urban	19.0%	80.0%	1.0%
	Rural	8.9%	88.9%	2.2%
Monthly income (Rp)	> 150 000	18.7%	79.9%	1.4%
	< 150 000	8.7%	89.3%	2.0%
Prenatal care				
Location	Urban	49.4%	45.3%	5.3%
	Rural	56.1%	35.6%	7.3%
Monthly income (Rp)	> 150 000	49.5%	44.1%	7.3%
	< 150 000	55.9%	36.2%	7.9%
Inpatient services				
Location	Urban	56.3%	43.7%	
	Rural	65.9%	34.1%	
Monthly income (Rp)	> 150 000	59.0%	41.0%	
	< 150 000	66.2%	33.8%	

High percentage of utilization of private delivery services mostly attributed to use of traditional birth attendants.
Rp 150 000 is equal to US$ 70 (1995 exchange rate).
[a]Others include self-medication, no treatment, or more than one type of provider.
Source: Malek (1992).

11.3.2   Ambulatory care

The Susenas data on health-seeking behavior allow calculation of the number of sick people utilizing different kinds of providers, both public and private. Table 11.2 presents information about utilization expressed in percentages to allow comparisons among providers.

Private providers play a substantial role in the provision of ambulatory care, comparable to that of public providers. Doctors and paramedics are the two most commonly used providers. Table 11.2 demonstrates urban–rural and high–low-income differences of utilization between public and private providers. It shows that urban and richer families tend to use private providers more than rural and poorer families.

11.3.3   Prenatal care

For prenatal care services, a substantial role is played by private providers, although in total they provide fewer services than public providers (see Table 11.2).

Private midwives are preferred among private providers although their role is less than that of the public health centers. Despite concerted efforts to train TBAs in maternity care and to make them available in villages, their role in providing prenatal care is limited.

11.3.4 Delivery care

Unlike prenatal care services, most deliveries are performed by private providers. Eighty-nine per cent of all deliveries were assisted by private providers. TBAs played a major role, performing 58 per cent of deliveries. This evidence is supported by other studies conducted in 1994–95, during which time thousands of village midwives were already in place. One study revealed that 85 to 90 per cent of deliveries were assisted by TBAs although 80 to 85 per cent of prenatal care was provided by village midwives.

Patterns of delivery care utilization between urban and rural and between higher and lower incomes are consistent: all families used private providers more than public providers (see Table 11.2).

11.3.5 Inpatient care

More than one-third of inpatient care in the country took place in private hospitals and other private facilities (such as maternity clinics with beds for inpatient care). This is consistent with the fact that 30 per cent of the hospital beds in Indonesia are in private hospitals.

Forty-four per cent of urban people used private hospitals, as opposed to 34 per cent of rural people. A similar pattern is evident with respect to income levels. As shown in Table 11.2, 41 per cent of the richer segment of the population used private hospitals compared to 34 per cent of the lower-income group.

11.4 HEALTH SECTOR REFORM

Despite the government's success in establishing a sizable network of health services, current demand for high-quality medical care exceeds the government's capacity to supply services. Given this situation, a set of policies has been developed during the last 10 years. Although each of the policy initiatives was developed separately, they were actually a package of interrelated policies directed toward more equitable and accessible services with improved quality. As a whole, the policies also promote a greater role for private health development in Indonesia.

11.4.1 Major policy initiatives

Major policy initiatives include the contracting of doctors and midwives (see sections 11.2.1.1 and 11.2.1.4).

11.4.1.1 Resource mobilization through prepayment systems. Prepayment systems are seen as mechanisms to mobilize more resources from nongovernment sources. Seventy per cent of health expenditure in Indonesia comes from private sources, in the form of out-of-pocket payments (75 per cent), employer expenditures (19 per cent), and prepayment mechanisms (6 per cent).

Currently only about 11 per cent of the almost 200 million population is covered by the prepayment system. The growth of the prepayment system has been very slow in Indonesia, despite systematic efforts undertaken since the early 1980s to stimulate the system. The reasons for low coverage include high subsidies in government health facilities that do not create a high financial risk to the population; the extended family system that works as a kind of insurance; and weakness in health insurance infrastructures to promote and market health insurance products (Gani, 1990).

Low coverage of health insurance has created a certain amount of bad debt in health service facilities, especially hospitals. To some extent, it also limits the growth of private provision of health services.

In 1992 the government enacted three separate laws related to health prepayment plans. It is expected that the three laws will stimulate the development of the prepayment system as a way of mobilizing more health resources.

Private health insurance programs are also expanding. PT. Askes, a state company managing health insurance for 15 million government employees and retirees, and their families, is now trying to expand its market to nongovernment employees. It started systematic marketing in 1993 to attract workers in the private sector. Several private firms in Central Java and around 80 per cent of the private firms on Batam Island have joined PT. Askes.

11.4.1.2 Decentralization and integrated planning and budgeting. To reduce problems arising from the top-down and fragmented health planning and budgeting, the Department of Health has taken an initiative called "Integrated Health Planning and Budgeting". This new system was implemented beginning in the 1993–94 fiscal year.

In 1994, the Ministry of Internal Affairs decentralized, giving more autonomy to the district level. Under the new policy, the District Health Office has more power to execute Integrated Health Planning and Budgeting. With this autonomy, there is more possibility for the health office to explore and implement users' fee adjustments in hospitals and health centers.

11.4.1.3 Restricting new public hospital construction and promoting the private sector. Hospitals absorb 35 per cent of the total government health budget. This led to the government's decision to adopt the policy restraining new hospital construction at least until the year 2000. To meet increasing demand for hospitals, the government has also adopted a policy to deregulate hospital investment. Since the adoption of this policy in 1989, there has been a significant increase in the number of hospitals and hospital beds owned by the private sector, by both domestic and foreign investors.

11.4.1.4 The Unit Swadana hospital. "Unit Swadana" is the government policy to allow public facilities to adjust prices according to market demand, and to retain and utilize their revenue (Ministry of Finance, 1992). It is described in detail in section 11.5.

11.4.1.5 Assuring access for the less fortunate. An important priority of the government is to assure access for the poor. Many of the policies described above have had, to a certain extent, a negative impact on the poor. This is especially true of users' fees and the promotion of private providers. To offset these negative effects, there are three interrelated policies being implemented in many areas of Indonesia.

The first is promoting and intensifying the development of the Community Health Financing Scheme, commonly known as "Dana Sehat" (Health Fund). Dana Sehat collects contributions from its members to be used to pay for health services whenever any of its members suffers an illness. The size of the contribution varies from one Dana Sehat to another and is determined collectively by the Dana Sehat members.

The second is the national policy to empower families through the provision of "Welfare Saving". The initial amount is Rp 2000 (a little less than $1), given free by the government as initial savings for families in the villages. This program is funded by large national businesses (conglomerates). Beginning in 1995, the firms agreed to contribute 2 per cent of their profits for this "family welfare" movement. This movement will have a significant impact on village economic activities. Empowerment of family economies will improve their ability to pay the Dana Sehat contribution or health service fees. This policy will also strengthen the implementation of other policies such as Unit Swadana in health centers and hospitals, and the placement of family doctors in subdistricts and midwives in villages as private providers of health services.

The third policy related to assuring accessibility is the provision of free health cards to poor families, a program that started in 1993. All poor families are eligible for the health cards. The head of the village is in charge of distributing them in collaboration with the staff of the health centers.

11.4.2 Impact of the reforms

The reforms described above were conceptualized to achieve normative objectives in health development. As summarized in Table 11.3, each policy contributes to specific objectives.

The reforms described above are interdependent. The success of retaining doctors and midwives in their workplaces after their contracts expire is influenced by the community's ability to pay for services. The community's capacity, in turn, is dependent on the success of prepayment systems and family economic empowerment. The implementation of Unit Swadana for district hospitals and health centers is influenced by the capacity of the district health office to implement Integrated Health Planning and Budgeting, in which fee adjustments are included. Fee adjustment is dependent on the ability to pay. The concept of the Unit Swadana

Table 11.3. Impact of Health Policy Reforms on Health Objectives.

Health policy reform	Objectives					
	Improved equity	Expansion of PHC	Improved quality of care	Sustainability of health program	Reduced public spending	Mobilization of non-government resources
Contract doctors	+++	++++	++	+	+	NA
Contract midwives	++++	+++++	+++	+	+	NA
Jaminan Pemeliharaan Kesehatan Masyarakat	++	+++	++	+	+ and −	++++
International Health Planning and Budgeting	++	++	+	++	NA	+
Restraint of growth of public hospitals	+?	+	+++	+	+++	+++
Promotion of private hospital growth	−	−	+++	?	NA	+++
Unit Swadana hospital	+	+	++++	++	+	+++
Family empowerment	++++	++++	+	+	NA	++++

NA, not applicable; +, positive impact; −, negative impact.

hospital should therefore be seen as an integral part of the holistic health sector reform in Indonesia.

11.5 THE UNIT SWADANA ("SELF-SUSTAINING") HOSPITAL

"Swadana" is a Sanskrit word literally meaning self-financed. The name is used to represent the government policy of deregulating facilities for public services such as education and health. The policy was enacted through a presidential decree in 1991. One of the primary features of this decree is the decision to facilitate public hospital autonomy through their ability to generate, retain, and utilize their revenues through a specific planning and budgeting process (Department of Internal Affairs, 1993). With financial autonomy, the hospitals are able to operate like private hospitals in improving their efficiency and quality, while still promoting social equity.

11.5.1 Rationale

In the early years after Independence, faced with an inadequate health infrastructure and insufficient number of health providers, the government took responsibility for providing all medical services. During those years, individual and household incomes were low and the private health sector was underdeveloped.

The situation has changed, especially during the last 25 years. As noted above, demographic and epidemiological changes have created greater demands for more modern and sophisticated medical services. With the government's allocation of only 2.5 per cent of budget for the health sector, demand has exceeded the government's ability to provide the necessary subsidies. Therefore, ways must be found to maximize the effective use of both public and private resources and to reduce the dependency of the entire population on government financing and provision of health services. This includes promoting private investment in hospital services, as well as private financing of public hospitals.

Swadana hospitals were also needed to compensate for deficiencies in the management and organization of government hospitals. Hospital management did not have the autonomy and flexibility to improve hospital efficiency and quality. Hospital budgets came from different sources. The planning for use of funds from multiple sources had been fragmented and hospital managers lacked the authority to consolidate them. Moreover, there were no functioning committees on quality assurance in most public hospitals.

11.5.2 Description

11.5.2.1 Objectives. The primary objective of the Unit Swadana hospital is to give greater autonomy and flexibility to public hospitals (Department of Health, 1995) so that they can:

- Promote social equity and accessibility for all segments of the population
- Improve the quality of medical services

- Increase hospital efficiency through optimal resource utilization
- Retain hospital revenues and utilize these revenues for hospital operations, including staff incentives and
- Reduce government subsidies through users' fees (the saved amount to be utilized for promotive and preventive care).

11.5.2.2 Characteristics. The special characteristics of the Unit Swadana hospital are summarized in Table 11.4, and described as follows.

Promoting social equity and improving accessibility. The Unit Swadana hospital is directed toward promoting social equity and improving accessibility to the general population regardless of the ability to pay. This is done by developing the hospital's capacity to capture demand from affluent community members and cross-subsidizing those who are less fortunate. Cross-subsidy for the poor can be achieved within the pricing structure. It is clear, therefore, that profit maximization is not the objective of the Unit Swadana hospital.

Revenue retention. Under the 1991 presidential decree, the Unit Swadana hospital is allowed to retain and utilize its revenues. Revenues are to be used to improve hospital facilities and services and may not be invested or otherwise diverted to uses that do not directly provide care (Ministry of Finance, 1992). There are certain procedures that must be followed. The hospital has to make projections of its revenue for the coming fiscal year. The projected or expected amount is then proposed in a separate budget plan called "Daftar Rencana Kegiatan" (DRK), an activity-based budget list (Department of Internal Affairs, 1993).

In the DRK, there are three broad categories of budget items with respect to the use of the hospital revenues: (1) operational activities related to the production of hospital services; (2) hospital maintenance activities; and (3) a program for human resources development in the respective hospital. In the last category, the hospital can make a plan for increasing staff incentives, up to a maximum of 35 per cent of total hospital revenues. Thus, the Unit Swadana concept provides a mechanism to motivate staff to increase hospital revenues through quality improvement.

Table 11.4. Characteristics of Unit Swadana Hospitals.

Structure	Operational functions	Outcomes
Human resources investment and development Investment in equipment and technology Organizational change	Accounting system Costing, pricing cross-subsidy Revenue retention Quality assurance Marketing	Equity and accessibility Quality of care Efficiency Cost recovery

Marketing. In order to be financially self-sustaining, the Unit Swadana hospital has to generate sufficient demand for its services. The ability of the hospital to capture this demand is very much dependent on quality improvement and marketing strategies. Some ethical issues arise in regard to marketing hospital services, such as whether it is acceptable for the hospital to advertise prices or merely advertise the type of services available and hours of availability.

Marketing is a systematic program of building a positive image, undertaken by all hospital staff. Staff hospitality, cleanliness of the hospital, promptness in serving clients, and conformity to standard medical procedures are important elements of conveying a positive image to all clients, including regulatory bodies, financing agencies, and the general population.

Quality assurance. Revenue retention, incentives for hospital staff, and the establishment of a quality assurance (QA) committee are some strategies used for improving quality. Other strategies include adopting quality control circles (QCC) and the total quality management (TQM) approaches.

Even more important is the formulation of standards for medical procedures. The Department of Health, in collaboration with the Indonesian Medical Association, has formulated standards for 100 medical procedures. The work is still continuing to formulate standards for other procedures. However, since QA within the Unit Swadana concept is seen as a total improvement in the production of medical care in the hospital, it must also include nonmedical aspects, such as cleanliness.

Accounting system. Financial management in public hospitals uses a cash basis accounting system. However, this does not provide the data needed for a thorough cost analysis, especially on the cost of investment. Since cost analysis and unit cost-based pricing are essential in Unit Swadana operations, an accrual accounting system has been introduced. Conversion from cash basis to accrual accounting is an important process in the development of Unit Swadana hospitals (Stoeko, 1994).

Costing and pricing of services. Improved accounting systems will allow for a more accurate cost analysis of Swadana hospitals. The analysis produces estimates of the total cost and the breakdown of the cost into components, such as investment, operational, and maintenance costs. Such cost information, if it is made available regularly, can be utilized as a basis for cost containment.

Cost analysis can also produce the unit cost, which can be used for price determination. Guidelines for pricing Swadana hospital services have been made. These include unit costs, cost recovery, cross-subsidization, and hospital financial requirements as the basis for price determination. Unit cost information is also useful in evaluating the size of subsidies given to hospital users.

Human resources development. In order to capture the growing demand for better-quality hospital services, Swadana hospitals may have to recruit new staff (such as medical specialists, qualified nurses, and support staff, including medical equipment operators). Although the Unit Swadana hospital is subject to the national policy of zero growth for personnel, it is allowed to recruit its own staff as long as it has sufficient resources to pay their salaries.

For the Swadana hospital to operate like a private business entity, it needs skilled employees in data processing, marketing, accounting and financing, pricing, and QA procedures. Staff training thus becomes more important in the Swadana hospital.

Investment. The Unit Swadana hospital may need to open new medical services, construct new facilities, or procure new equipment. Decisions for these investments must be approved by the local government in the case of regional hospitals and by the MOH in the case of MOH hospitals. Investment in building and equipment can be done as a joint venture with private investors. This strategy helps resolve problems related to the government's policy to restrict new investment in public hospitals.

Organizational changes. All of the characteristics described above highlight strategic management functions, or even create new functions, essential in the operation of the Unit Swadana hospital. The organizational units that should be created or strengthened to perform or absorb the essential functions are committees on QA, financial management, medical records and hospital information, marketing, and hospital planning. The functions of each unit, as well as the qualifications and job descriptions of the personnel in these units, have been specified by the Directorate General of Medical Services of the MOH.

11.5.3 Experiences

The implementation of the Unit Swadana concept was initiated by the Department of Health in 1991. It was first implemented in five vertical hospitals controlled by the Department of Health on a project basis. The project, which was supported by external funding, also organized seminars and workshops to disseminate the concept.

Implementation of Unit Swadana has been replicated in a number of regional hospitals. At first, a few regional hospital directors took the initiative to convert their own hospitals into Unit Swadana hospitals. In December 1995, the Ministry of Internal Affairs organized a national workshop to explore the feasibility of turning more regional hospitals into Unit Swadana. In some places, the principles of Unit Swadana have also been implemented in health centers.

The criteria used in choosing hospitals to be converted into Unit Swadana are (Department of Health, 1995):

- The hospital has demonstrated efficient performance for 3 consecutive years, as indicated by its bed occupancy rate, length of stay, and turnover interval
- Its cost recovery rate has reached a level of 50 per cent
- There is evidence of commitment from the hospital administration, especially the director
- There is evidence of commitment and support from the Ministry of Internal Affairs and the local government
- The community served by the hospital has the ability to pay for its own medical services as indicated by socioeconomic data in the region.

Currently there are 13 vertical and some 26 regional hospitals already implementing all or part of the concept. The performance of a sample of these hospitals will be described (Soeharsono, 1995). The impact of implementing the concept of the internal management and financing of these hospitals will be examined. The impact of Unit Swadana on the development of the private sector will also be explored, focusing on the role of the private sector in the provision and financing of health services.

The discussion in this section is based on data obtained from visits to two Unit Swadana hospitals in West Java: Tangerang and Sumedang hospitals. Interviews were conducted with the directors and the chiefs of units in these hospitals. In the district of Sumedang, interviews were also conducted with the head of the local government and the district health officer. Secondary data were also collected, and reports on Unit Swadana implementation in other hospitals were reviewed.

11.5.4   Impact of the Unit Swadana hospital

11.5.4.1 Impact on public hospital management and financing.   The implementation of Unit Swadana has led to improvements in the management and financing of the hospitals. These improvements will be described in terms of cost analysis and rational pricing, inventory management, financial management and accounting, and hospital financing.

Cost analysis and rational pricing. Under Unit Swadana, public hospitals have become more cost-conscious in their operations and they have developed their own capacity to perform cost analysis. This information helps the hospital management to monitor cost behavior and set up a strategy for cost control.

As indicated above, cost analysis also produces estimates of the actual unit costs of various services. Most Unit Swadana hospitals use the unit cost information for bargaining for more rational payments from insurance companies and are now demanding price adjustments based on full unit costs.

Previously, regional hospitals had to undergo a long process of negotiation with the local house of representatives to obtain approval for price adjustments. With unit cost information, the process has been much faster. This has been the experience of four hospitals in East Kalimantan and West Nusatenggara provinces when, in 1995, they proposed new prices for their services.

Inventory management. As investment cost is an important element in cost analysis, Unit Swadana hospitals were forced to establish good inventory systems. As observed in Pasar Rebo Hospital in Jakarta and Tangerang and Sumedang hospitals in West Java, each unit in the hospital compiled a complete inventory of all investment items. The information includes the name of the investment item, factory name, year of procurement, and purchase price. This information makes it easier to calculate the investment cost of the item.

Financial management and accounting. Since the Unit Swadana hospital has to prepare a separate budget plan on the use of its revenues, the hospital management now has the authority to exercise principles of good financial management. This authority also allows the hospital management to shift funds from one item to another and to determine the size of a budget allocation, which was not possible before the Swadana policy. For example, determining the size and distribution of incentives among medical and nonmedical staff in Sumedang Hospital was done collectively in a workshop involving all hospital staff.

The implementation of an accrual accounting system is another improvement in the Unit Swadana hospital. However, due to the fact that the hospitals still receive fragmented allocations, they continue to maintain the old cash basis system. Personnel in the accounting unit of the hospital stated that using two accounting systems is rather inefficient.

Hospital financing. Hospital revenue is a function of price and utilization. Data from the Unit Swadana hospitals indicated that utilization did not diminish with changes in prices. Consequently, revenues will increase significantly. As presented in Table 11.5, the hospitals maintained their bed occupancy rate after they were turned into Unit Swadana. A sharp increase in total revenues was also demonstrated. With increased revenues, the hospitals were able to increase their allocation for operations, including staff incentives. Of the total revenue, 70 per cent was allocated for operational costs and 30 per cent for staff incentives. Distribution of incentives varies between hospitals. In Sumedang, 55 per cent of the total incentives was given to medical personnel and the remaining 45 per cent to paramedical and nonmedical staff.

In Tangerang, this achievement impressed the local government authorities, who, in response to increased revenues and improved quality of health care, allocated new capital investments. The local government has funded construction of a building for emergency care (ICU/ICCU) and a polyclinic. Water treatment and incinerator plants have also been constructed.

Table 11.5. Performance of Selected Hospitals before and after Implementation of the Unit Swadana Hospital Model.

Fiscal year	1990–91	1991–92	1992–93	1993–94	1994–95
Tangerang					
Bed occupancy rate (%)	75.0%	73.3%	74.5%	76.7%	74.6%
Revenue (× Rp 1000)	2 100 000	3 200 000	3 400 000	4 000 000	4 800 000
Revenue increase (%)		52.4%	6.3%	17.6%	20.0%
Sumedang					
Bed occupancy rate (%)	—	—	76.7%	84.0%	81.8%
Revenue (× Rp 1000)	786 947	904 869	1 067 346	1 845 695	2 420 020
Revenue increase (%)		14.9%	17.9%	72.9%	31.1%
Kudus					
Bed occupancy rate (%)	84.0%	80.0%	87.0%	82.0%	73.0%
Revenue (× Rp 1000)	932 406	1 106 146	1 365 368	1 992 549	2 328 909
Revenue increase (%)		18.6%	23.4%	45.9%	16.9%

The three hospitals were converted into Unit Swadana hospitals in 1993–94.

11.5.4.2 Impact on equity. As far as equity is concerned, the most crucial issue is whether converting a public hospital into a Unit Swadana hospital will exclude the poor from the hospital services. Data from the Tangerang hospital demonstrate that equity was maintained during the implementation of the Unit Swadana concept.

In Indonesia, a hospital bed is classified as VIP, class-I, class-II, or class-III, depending on the level of services received by the patient and the corresponding cost. In some hospitals, the subsidy given to users of VIP beds is much higher than that given to the users of class-III beds. In the Unit Swadana hospital, such problems can be corrected by implementing cross-subsidization. The prices charged for VIP and class-I beds are set at a level higher than their unit cost. The profit generated from VIP and class-I beds is used to subsidize class-III beds. According to the guidelines on pricing for Swadana hospitals, the price for class-III should cover only the nonsalary component of its unit cost (for example, food, drugs, and supplies).

As revenue generation is an important feature of the Unit Swadana concept, the tendency is to invest in expanding VIP and class-I inpatient beds. To avoid the hospital neglecting its social function, the MOH guidelines on the Unit Swadana hospital have determined a desired composition of the number of beds in each class: 50 per cent in class-III (minimum) and 50 per cent in VIP and class-I and class-II (maximum). This composition is considered sufficient to allow the hospital to generate revenue from VIP, class-I, and class-II beds and to use the revenue for efficiency and quality improvement, as well as cross-subsidizing those treated in class-III beds.

Assuming that class-III beds were used by the lower-income group, data in Table 11.6 show that the bed occupancy rate remained at a high level after the concept was introduced in 1993–94. The 9 per cent of hospital billings which were bad debt in 1994–95 may indicate that low-income-level people did use the facility, if it is assumed that most of the bad debt was incurred by the poor.

In Sumedang, the head of the district government stated that the exclusion of the poor can be avoided by developing a prepayment system. Therefore, he has taken an active role in supporting the development of Dana Sehat in the district. Through his authority, he has asked subdistrict and village heads in the district to help health offices and centers develop Dana Sehat.

Table 11.6. Bed Occupancy Rate by Inpatient Service Category, Tangerang Hospital.

Fiscal year	1990–91	1991–92	1992–93	1993–94	1994–95
VIP	62.9%	56.6%	66.4%	73.3%	81.3%
Class-I	69.2%	70.5%	76.8%	80.9%	84.6%
Class-II	80.9%	74.7%	72.7%	69.6%	78.3%
Class-III	74.5%	71.4%	72.3%	77.4%	81.5%
ICU	41.8%	52.7%	59.9%	68.7%	64.5%
Perinatal	75.5%	87.6%	80.5%	97.0%	62.6%
Total	74.8%	73.2%	74.5%	76.7%	78.3%

VIP, Luxurious rooms, most expensive; Class-I, private rooms; Class-II, semiprivate rooms, least expensive; Class-III, rooms for patients who cannot pay; ICU, intensive care unit.
Source: Tangerang Hospital Annual Statisics (1995). Unpublished.

More interesting is the amount of subsidies paid by Sumedang Hospital for various types of users (government employees, the poor, users of free health cards, and bad debt). Before the hospital was converted into a Unit Swadana hospital, the amount of subsidy expenditure was Rp 42.8 million. After its conversion in 1993–94, the hospital spent Rp 182.6 million. This amount was sustained in the following years.

11.5.4.3 Impact on quality

Improvement in human resources. Since the Unit Swadana hospital is allowed to recruit its own staff, in Sumedang Hospital, the director recruited medical doctors who had finished their 3-year contract working in government health centers. The hospital also recruited nurses and provided fellowships for postgraduate training in hospital administration for two of its staff.

Improving hospital performance through the QCC approach. The QCC approach has been implemented in Pasar Rebo Hospital in Jakarta since it was converted into a Unit Swadana hospital in 1992. Eighteen quality circle teams were established. The teams meet once or twice each week after work for several hours. Many quality problems have been solved as a result. One remarkable success was an improvement in the cleanliness of the hospital (Haryadi, 1994). The principles and methods of QCC and TQM have also been implemented in other Swadana hospitals, such as Klaten and Kudus (both in Central Java).

Patient satisfaction. Implementation of Unit Swadana in Sumedang Hospital resulted in improvements in patient satisfaction. This assertion is based on patient satisfaction surveys conducted every year since 1993. The surveys revealed improvements in patients' perceptions of and satisfaction with cleanliness, medical and inpatient services, and administrative services. These improvements are apparently attributable to increased availability of services and the positive attitude of hospital staff since the Swadana implementation.

11.5.4.4 Impact on private sector development.

The conversion of public hospitals into Unit Swadana has had a great impact on the development of the private sector in the provision and financing of health services. In general, the growing number of Unit Swadana hospitals has made the market for hospital services more competitive. Most private hospitals in Indonesia, especially those established during the 1980s and 1990s, were known to cater to the upper segment of the population concentrated in urban areas. Previously, public hospitals were perceived by this segment as having low quality and serving primarily the poor. Gradually this image is changing with the growth of Unit Swadana hospitals.

Private investors now see the Unit Swadana hospitals as good opportunities for investment. For example, Tangerang Hospital, a district public hospital that converted to a Unit Swadana in 1993, attracted the attention of a private investor, who funded the construction of a new ward of 50 beds. General Electric has also invested in installing computed tomography scans and other high-technology medical equipment. The private sector has invested in several other Unit Swadana hospitals, mostly in equipment.

Unit Swadana has also affected the medical human resources in private hospitals. With better incentives and improved quality of medical facilities, public hospitals have more capacity to attract and retain medical specialists. This is the case with Tangerang Hospital. Despite competitive offers from surrounding modern private hospitals, medical specialists are inclined to work in Tangerang Hospital. This situation has stimulated private hospitals to find other ways of recruiting medical specialists. Some private hospitals attempt to recruit Indonesian doctors who work abroad. Other hospitals have begun investing in training for their own medical specialists.

11.6   CONCLUSION

It is obvious that the private sector has been playing a major role in the provision of health services in Indonesia. It is likely that the role of the private health sector will continue to grow rapidly. This is due primarily to two major government policies. The first is the policy to limit the number of public hospitals, allowing the private sector to capture the growing demand for hospital services. The second is the policy to contract doctors and midwives to serve in the public sector for a 3-year period, after which many go into private practice. These two policies will continue to be a strong impetus for the growth of this sector in Indonesia, at least until the year 2000.

These are just two of the many policies initiated by the government to develop more equitable and accessible services with improved quality. Unit Swadana, an integral part of comprehensive health sector reform, aims to give greater autonomy and flexibility to public sector health facilities.

The primary objectives of this policy are promoting equity and accessibility, quality of care, efficiency, and cost recovery. These objectives are to be achieved through revenue retention and strengthening specific management functions, including accounting systems, costing and pricing, quality assurance, and marketing. Certain investments are also implicit in the Unit Swadana concept, including human resources training and investment in equipment and technology.

As of 1995, the concept had been introduced in 13 central and 26 district hospitals. Based on documented reports and observations made in two Unit Swadana hospitals, the concept has indeed succeeded in increasing hospital revenue substantially. With additional revenues and flexibility in their utilization, Unit Swadana hospitals have also succeeded in improving their service quality. Most importantly, the Unit Swadana concept has not led to excluding the poor from using the hospitals.

The Unit Swadana policy has affected the development of the private sector. First, it has created more constraints by restricting medical specialists from working on a part-time basis in private hospitals. However, this situation will presumably stimulate the private sector to train its own medical specialists or secure medical specialists from elsewhere.

Second, the Unit Swadana has attracted private investors, both multinational and domestic, to invest in public hospitals. This phenomenon will speed the integration of the public and private health sectors. Theoretical discussion of whether there should be a public/private mix of health services is obsolete, as the discussion has shifted to what the composition of that mix should be.

Third, increased prices in the Unit Swadana have created awareness of higher financial risks among patients. This in turn has stimulated the development of prepayment systems, such as health insurance, managed care programs, and community health funds. Since these systems provide subsidized premiums to their members, the effect of Unit Swadana is therefore a more equitable subsidy than subsidies provided only at the point of service. This is because a cross-subsidy mechanism is inherent in the Unit Swadana concept.

REFERENCES

Akin, J., Birdsall, N., de Ferranti, D. (1987). *Financing Health Services in Developing Countries: An Agenda for Reform.* Washington, DC: World Bank.

Bureau of Planning, Ministry of Health. (1995). *Health Care Financing Reform in Indonesia.* Bangkok: WHO Intercountry Consultation on Health Care Financing Reform.

Department of Health. (1995). *Guidelines for Proposing and Managing the Vertical Unit Swadana Hospital.* Jakarta.

Department of Internal Affairs. (1993). *Ministry of Internal Affairs Decree on Financial Accountability of Regional Unit Swadana.* Jakarta.

Gani, A. (1990). Resources mobilization in the health sector. *Prisma* **19**(6).

Haryadi, A. (1994). *Hospital Quality Improvement: Experience in Pasar Rebo Hospital.* Denpasar: International Conference on Hospital Quality Improvement.

Jeffers, J. (1990). Supply, demand and socio-economic factors influencing health policies. *Prisma* **19**(6).

Malek, R. (1992). *Health Services based on 1990 National Socioeconomic Survey.* National Health Research Institute, Department of Health, Indonesia.

Ministry of Finance. (1992). *Guidelines for Unit Swadana.* Jakarta.

Soeharsono, A. (1995). *Role of Health Insurance in District Hospital Development*, National Workshop on Unit Swadana Hospital. Ministry of Internal Affairs, Mataram.

Stoeko, P. (1994). *Unit Swadana and the Swadanization Process of Government Hospitals.* Jakarta: Health Sector Financing Project, Department of Health. Unpublished working paper.

World Bank. (1987). Country study: Indonesia. *Health Planning and Budgeting.* Washington, DC: World Bank.

Part V
Conclusion

12

The Future of Health Sector Reform in Asia

WILLIAM NEWBRANDER

Health Economist, Management Sciences for Health

and

PATRICIA MOSER

Project Economist, Asian Development Bank

12.1 INTRODUCTION

Throughout the world, countries at all levels of the economic and political spectrum are undertaking health sector reform. Asia, with its strong and vibrant national economies, is no exception. The objectives of health sector reform are to bring about fundamental changes in the health system that will help meet national health objectives while making the system sustainable financially, organizationally, and politically. As the specific national objectives vary from country to country, so do the strategies each country adopts. The private health sector has a role to play no matter what strategies are adopted. The preceding chapters aptly illustrate these differing approaches and differing roles for the private sector.

Within its theme of the growth of the private sector in the context of health sector reform in Asia, this book has focused on the demand side, the supply side, and quality of care issues. These issues, including regulations, payment mechanisms, financing methods, and quality assessments, are interrelated. During medical transactions, they all affect the individual patient's experience and health outcomes, as well as impacting the country's health system in its totality. Thus they affect equity, efficiency, and quality of care whether the care is delivered by public or private providers.

This chapter presents a summary of the private health sector in Asia, as well as the key demand-side, supply-side, and quality issues. It highlights the key challenges for Asia in the future in each of those areas and concludes with some specific recommendations for action.

Private Health Sector Growth in Asia: Issues and Implications. Edited by W. Newbrander.
© 1997 John Wiley & Sons, Ltd.

12.2 THE PRIVATE HEALTH SECTOR IN ASIA

Significant progress has been made in improving the health status of many countries of Asia over the past two decades. However, countries must continue to cope with demographic changes due to population growth and aging; epidemiological challenges, with the increase of chronic diseases and the emergence of new diseases such as AIDS; and the rising expectations of the population for more and better health services.

While the countries of Asia vary in their levels of economic growth, income, education, urbanization, employment, and health care provision, they are generally committed to the goal of pluralism, involving both the public and private sectors in all elements of the economy and society. This attitude is reflected in the significant role of the private health sector in the health systems of most of the countries in the region.

In general, as countries' income levels have increased, national health expenditures have increased. This occurs because countries with growing economies tend to invest more in their health sectors. The means of financing health care vary from the socialized health systems (where the government finances health expenditure out of general tax revenues and operates many of the facilities) to those that have opted for private delivery, with a mix of public and private financing of health services.

The share of the private sector in total health expenditure is large and has been increasing with the strong economic growth of countries in the region. In general, the government accounts for between 22 and 51 per cent of a country's total national health expenditure in the six countries that are the focus of this book (see Table 12.1). When all the countries of the region are considered, the differences are more pronounced: from lows of 21.7 per cent in India and 22.0 per cent in Thailand to a high of 73.8 per cent in Japan in 1991. The median percentage of national health expenditure from public sources for 16 Asian countries was 48.8 per cent, while the mean percentage was 47.2 per cent. Social health insurance is taking on an increasingly major role in financing of health services, while private health insurance has remained relatively insignificant in the region (see Chapter 7, Table 7.1).

The government's proportion of total health expenditure will probably continue to decline in Asia, especially in those countries with lower growth rates. As the government's role in financing the health sector diminishes, its role in the design, operation, and provision of services in their health systems will change. Since the source of finance affects the type and location of services provided and their accessibility, changes in the source of finance may have important impacts on the progressiveness with which the health sector is financed and the equity with which its services are available to those in greatest need.

Provision of health services indicates a wide variation among the six countries in the public and private control of hospitals. Using data collected by the authors of the preceding chapters, Table 12.2 shows the range (30 to 95 per cent) for the percentage of private hospitals. The percentage range of private hospital beds is less dramatic: 22 to 77 per cent. These figures reflect the situation in most Asian countries, where the number of private hospitals is large but their size is small compared to that of public hospitals.

Patients from all economic strata have increasingly used private health facilities and providers, including private hospitals, physicians, traditional healers, and pharmacists.

Table 12.1. National Health Expenditure, Selected Countries, 1991.

Country	GDP per capita (US$)	National health expenditure (% GDP)	Per capita national health expenditure (US$)	Per cent expenditure from public sources
India	310	6.0	21	21.7
Indonesia	670	2.0	12	35.0
Korea	770	2.0	14	50.0
Philippines	1840	5.0	73	22.0
Thailand	6790	6.6	377	40.9
Vietnam	NA	NA	NA	50.8

NA, not applicable.
Sources: World Bank. (1993). *World Development Report 1993: Investing in Health*. New York: Oxford University Press. World Bank. (1995). *Vietnam Poverty Assessment and Strategy*. Washington, DC: World Bank.

Table 12.2. Public and Private Hospitals and Beds, Various Years.

Country	Hospitals			Beds			
	No.	Public (%)	Private (%)	No.	Public (%)	Private (%)	Beds per 1000 pop.[a]
India (1992)	11 174	43	57	642 103	68	32	0.7
Indonesia (1994)	1039	58	42	116 847	68	32	0.7
Korea (1994)	650	5	95	124 597	23	77	3.0
Philippines (1993)	1632	33	67	71 865	50	50	1.3
Thailand (1993)	1188	70	30	108 368	78	22	1.6
Vietnam	NA	NA	NA	NA	NA	NA	NA

NA, not available.
[a]Data from World Bank (1993). *World Development Report 1993: Investing in Health*. New York: Oxford University Press.

Data presented in Chapter 9 (see Figure 9.1 and Table 9.5) and Chapter 11 (see Table 11.2) illustrate the rapid growth in private sector provision of services in the region. The consumer's perception of the relative advantages of the private sector, with respect to quality of care, availability of services and drugs, amenities, location, and waiting time, helps explain this change in utilization patterns, as Mongkolsmai pointed out (Chapter 6).

It is in this context that the countries of the region are seeking to find those strategies and solutions that will allow them to use the public and private sources of financing and providers to address demand-side, supply-side, and quality of care issues.

12.3   DEMAND-SIDE ISSUES: FINANCING AND HEALTH INSURANCE

12.3.1   *Public sector financing and private sector growth*

Governments throughout the region suffer from a lack of financing for the level and quality of services demanded by various groups. Hence, many believe the limited public funds should be better targeted toward increasing the quality of preventive and promotive services and providing personal health services on behalf of the poor. To do this, some argue that governments should control or even stop the expansion of tertiary facilities until basic minimum levels of services are available to the entire population. However, many countries prefer seeking other ways to mobilize additional resources for health service delivery rather than constraining the growth of hospitals.

The private sector is growing and is filling in many of the gaps the public system has been unable to fill. In general, the growth of the private sector has been good in terms of providing more services than governments can afford to make available, increasing the level of investment in the health sector, and upgrading the quality of health services. Concerns exist, however, about whether such growth is beneficial for achieving national health objectives. Experience has shown that demand for curative health services from those who are able to pay may skew the health system away from promoting national welfare and meeting the needs of the population in general.

12.3.2   Options for financing

Some of the immediate options considered for the financing of national health objectives are user fees and national health insurance (NHI).

User fees charged at government facilities are an important source of revenue that could be used to increase the quality of public services. User fees must be scaled or exemption mechanisms must be in place so the fees do not create an access barrier for the poor.

National health insurance programs are often the best vehicles for promoting equity, efficiency, and quality of care. However, these programs are extremely complicated to develop, organize, and manage. Some of the issues to be addressed in the development of NHI are decentralization of programs, voluntary versus compulsory enrollment, quality, costs, benefits or types of services covered, coverage of the population, financing, and incentives for providers. If universal coverage is the ultimate objective, compulsory participation is required in order to avoid adverse selection, and keep the rich from opting out of NHI programs to avoid having to subsidize the poor. Many countries, such as Thailand and the Philippines, already have several social financing programs in various stages of development and implementation.

12.3.3   The future

In order to finance health services adequately, governments must either increase their sources of financing (for example, through increased health budgets, increased user fees, expanded private health insurance or health maintenance organizations, or expanded programs of NHI and community financing); find ways to reduce the costs of health delivery systems through increased efficiency and effectiveness; or relinquish to the private health sector responsibility for the delivery of health services in segments of the market. Combinations of all of these approaches are possible. A number of actions and priorities with respect to financing are required of countries seeking to undertake meaningful health sector reform. These include:

- Policy-makers need to identify appropriate roles for public sector financing in the health sector, such as increasing equity or correcting market failures

- Public spending must be rationally targeted, unnecessary subsidies must be eliminated, and public facilities need to increase their efficiency
- If NHI is adopted, such programs should start modestly and evolve gradually toward universal coverage. During this time, measures to control fraud and abuse can be developed and experience can be gained in managing such programs effectively
- Other forms of insurance that promote cost containment, such as managed care, should incorporate concern for the poor, people in rural areas, and other disenfranchised groups and translate it into effective programs that relieve the burden of financing on these target groups
- Information sharing and policy exchange between countries in the region about health financing is essential. Appropriate solutions for the health financing problems of different countries need to be identified. This would help countries benefit from the results of research on and evaluation and monitoring of health financing and health insurance in other countries of the region.

12.4 SUPPLY-SIDE ISSUES: PAYMENT MECHANISMS AND REGULATION

Chapters 7, 8, and 9 offer information on as well as analysis of supply-side issues. Given the diversity of the Asian countries, there is considerable variation in how they deal with payment methods and regulation.

12.4.1 Payment methods

Disenchantment with the results obtained from public salaried health workers and the need to expand resources has led many countries to experiment with alternative methods of provider payment for the public sector. Recognition of accelerating growth in the costs of services in the private sector, particularly the growing claim on social insurance resources where such schemes exist, has also led governments to review payment methods and provider incentives in the private sector. In both sectors, the common beginning point for nonbudgetary payments is in the form of fees for services paid by clients directly to providers.

For the public sector, fee-for-service payments are usually in the form of user fees that cover part of service costs. This is especially the case in lower-income countries, for several reasons. First, it increases resources with little effect on government budgets. Second, it appears to be administratively simple, although this is often not the case. Third, it is appealing to providers as a means of achieving fee-for-service payment. However, user fees for public services, or any method of fee-for-service, tend to create access barriers for the poor. In addition to equity issues, fees for services also have the potential of burdening the ill with the costs of health sector development.

Another issue is retention of fees by public sector institutions providing services. Most of the Asian countries have moved away from the public financing norms that required government-generated revenues to be remitted to the treasury or other national financial institutions. This allows providers to keep and utilize these funds.

As shown in Chapter 11, when revenues are retained by institutions that have discretion in their use, user fees can actually improve equity and efficiency in the financing of health services, provided appropriate exemptions are made for the poor.

As user fees become increasingly important as a method of financing for the health sector, the need for insurance mechanisms to spread the risk of high financial costs associated with an illness also increases. However, fee-for-service payment methods coupled with increased financing in the sector, either through insurance mechanisms or improved incomes, tends to escalate the costs of service provision by removing financial barriers to demand for and use of services. As a result, the quantity, as well as the intensity of services used, increases. In many countries in Asia, both private and public sector financiers are experimenting with different provider payment mechanisms to slow the cost increases and improve efficiencies in the health sector. Countries with significant health insurance coverage or higher incomes may have attained adequate resources for the sector but now need to use alternative payment methods to improve allocative and productive efficiencies.

Provider payment methods create bargaining power for both payers and providers. Payers can make demands on providers when offering new incentives. However, providers may also band together and exert pressure on payers. For example, in Malaysia, the National Heart Center refused to accept lump-sum payments for treating the poor, instead demanding and receiving fee-for-service payments. The incentives of a fee-for-service system tend to increase the quantity of services demanded and used and the intensity of those services. As a result, lower-income countries are usually concerned with improving the provider payment system and getting it to work efficiently.

12.4.2   Regulation

All health systems are subject to various market failures and abuse. This creates the need for regulation to control these problems. Regulation is especially important when governments are undertaking privatization. However, governments often lack the capacity to initiate and maintain an effective regulatory system that has legislative authority, strong organizational structures, and the ability to monitor utilization and quality of health services. If new regulatory efforts are to be launched, it is important to ensure that there are significant benefits to be gained in terms of national health goals.

12.4.3   The future

Greater attention must be paid to payment mechanisms and the incentives associated with them as well as to medical and health regulations. Existing payment mechanisms and regulations need to be revised to reduce redundancy, to make them more practical, and to eliminate unintended perverse incentives for providers. Serious attempts must be made to provide adequate budgets and personnel to properly enforce regulations. The role of the private health sector in revising health laws and regulations, developing new ones, and working to enforce them is an item on the policy agenda in most countries in the region. A number of actions and priorities related to paying providers and regulation are required of countries seeking to undertake meaningful health sector reform. These include:

• Provider payments should be linked to health policy priorities and must be comparable to other sectors. To be effective in changing provider behavior, payments must comprise a significant proportion of providers' total earnings
• There is a need for more experimentation, exchange, and collaboration in the Asian region as regards regulation
• Nonregulatory means of influencing private sector behavior should be reviewed. For example, further study should be made of joint investments, such as the one in India where the government has invested jointly with private investors to construct an urban hospital. In exchange for its investment, the government can claim a certain percentage of beds for poor patients, with all recurrent costs borne by the hospital from total earnings.

12.5 QUALITY OF CARE ISSUES

12.5.1 Need for consumer education

Quality of care has drawn extensive interest recently for several reasons. Ineffective care often yields both poor health outcomes and waste of resources. Moreover, continued perceptions of poor quality can undermine the credibility of the government health system. The problem is complicated by the fact that the consumer is unable to judge many aspects of quality and is dependent on the provider to make critical choices. These problems are magnified when the private sector is increasingly responsible for the production and distribution of health services. Thus it is important to educate consumers about what they should expect from providers. Strategies to educate consumers can go a long way toward making market distribution of health services more effective.

12.5.2 Assessment of quality

There are different dimensions of quality, each of which implies different measures and responses. Individual encounters involve both clinical quality, based on technical criteria, and interpersonal quality, based on patients' perceptions of and responses to their interactions with providers. This latter dimension will be affected by time and resource constraints. Quality can also refer to institutional or facility attributes and ultimately to attributes of the system. In general, an appropriate level of quality is considered to be care that aims to do good, avoids harm, and maintains the balance of health in individuals.

The means for assessing quality must overcome the tendency to focus solely on the provider or supply side of the experience, as is the case with many currently used measures. Patient or user responses also need to be considered in the assessment. Continuity of assessment is important, both to provide a clearer picture of the overall dimensions of quality and to develop expanded capacity within the system for self-monitoring and performance improvement. If such assessment and monitoring are to be effective, the results of quality assessments need to be shared with the public. This is particularly important where public and private providers are competing for users. By making the assessment of quality part of the consumer decision, some of the limitations of market distributions can be overcome. This, of course, accentuates the need for development of cost-effective and valid measures of quality through scientific development and testing of indicators.

Accreditation and continuous quality assurance activities appear to be the most widely used means for ensuring quality of care in the private sector. However, the private and public sectors must be subject to the same quality criteria to avoid double standards. Professional associations have an important role to play in establishing and maintaining quality standards. They can define standards, provide training, and assess qualifications. They are less effective at direct assessment, monitoring the process of care, or responding to poor performance. One caution is that the potential role of professional bodies to carry out some essential elements of the quality review and assessment process must be limited to ensure they are not co-opted by the process.

12.5.3   The future

The quality of care delivered (viewed in the light of technical characteristics and consumer perceptions) lies at the heart of the effectiveness of the provision of services. Regardless of what policy decisions are made as to the appropriate mix of public and private sectors, both public and private sectors must work together to deliver a level of quality that is medically effective and is acceptable to consumers. A number of actions and priorities with respect to improving quality of care are required of countries seeking to undertake meaningful health sector reform. These include:

- Increase efforts to identify cost-saving quality improvements
- Increase capacity building in quality improvement, including training, intercountry visits, and national and regional institutional resources
- Undertake pilot studies of quality improvement, including improved methods of information collection, regulation and enforcement
- Facilitate regional and subregional meetings on quality and private/public sector interactions for exchanging experiences and learning from other countries in the region.

12.6   MOVING TO ACTION

Private sector growth poses a complicated set of strengths, weaknesses, opportunities, and threats to the achievement of health sector goals in each country in Asia. The region's countries are diverse: they range from low to high levels of income; the mix of public and private sector delivery and financing varies in each country; and the attitudes and political approaches to deal with the rapid development of the private health sector differ. In general, the private health sector in all countries of the region is growing significantly in size and complexity. This growth has been triggered by increasing levels of income, coupled with health insurance and other forms of collective financing arrangements.

In some countries, the private sector has already overtaken the public sector in size and importance in many areas of health service delivery, especially in the delivery of curative or personal health service delivery. Growth in the private sector opens up opportunities for countries to reappraise traditional ways of thinking. They can determine how the health service delivery and financing systems should be organized and operated in each country and what public and private sector mix is most appropriate for them to meet their specific national health sector goals.

There is a need for more research and sharing of experiences in terms of the growth and effects of private sector participation in the health sector. The role of government in the health sector is at the heart of public policy as it relates to health sector reform. Governments must have more information concerning the appropriate timing, rate of progress, and implications of changes in their roles. They also need information concerning formulation and development of appropriate policies and regulatory and incentive systems. As the countries of the region continue to develop, they will require assistance in designing and introducing the processes of research, monitoring, and evaluation that will inform them of the implications, results, and impact of policy initiatives (or lack of them) over time.

In order to meet these needs and to promote vigorous and desirable health sector reform in the future, the following recommendations are put forth. These six specific steps for action involve three levels: national, regional, and global (Table 12.3).

Table 12.3. Six Steps for Action at National, Regional, and Global Levels.

National
1. If it is to remain viable, the public sector as a provider of health services requires basic standards of quality to maintain its credibility and sufficient demand for its services. Improvements are necessary in financing methods, regulations, provider payment mechanisms, and quality of care
2. Within countries, the public and private sectors must collaborate to find appropriate mechanisms to make these improvements
3. The role of the public sector as a financier of health services needs to be firmly based on economic and political considerations, rather than historical precedent.
4. Additional information is needed on populations with low access to basic health services to target public resources appropriately so that equity goals are achieved efficiently

Regional
5. There is the need for countries to share information and experiences, test different models, and then facilitate change to bring about improved financing methods, regulations, provider payment mechanisms, and quality of care in the public and private sectors

Global
6. International organizations and multilateral and bilateral agencies should collaborate by providing technical assistance and financial aid and by supporting policy reviews and forums for sharing and disseminating information among countries about their experiences with health sector reform

---

Selected Bibliography

Akin, J., Birdsall, N., de Ferranti, D. (1987). *Financing Health Services in Developing Countries: An Agenda for Reform*. Washington, DC: World Bank.

Akin, J., Guilkey, D., Griffin, C., Popkin, B. (1985). *The Demand for Primary Health Services in the Third World*. Totowa, NJ: Rowman and Allenheld.

Barnum, H., Kutzin, J., Saxenian, H. (1995). *Incentives and Provider Payment Methods*. HRO Working Paper No. 5. Washington, DC: World Bank.

Bennett, S. (1992). Promoting the private sector: a review of developing country trends. *Health Policy and Planning*, **7**(2), 97–110.

Bennett, S., Tangcharoensathien, V. (1994). A shrinking state? Politics, economics and private health care in Thailand. *Public Administration and Development*, **14**, 1–17.

Bennett, S., Dakpallah, G., Garner, P., Gilson, L., Nittayaramphong, S., Zwi, A. (1994). Carrot and stick: state mechanisms to influence private provider behavior. *Health Policy and Planning*, **9**(1), 1–13.

Berman, P., Rannan-Eliya, R. (1993). *Factors Affecting the Development of Private Health Care Provision in Developing Countries*. Major Applied Research Paper No. 9. Bethesda, MD: Health Financing and Sustainability Project.

Berman, P., Hanson, K. (1994). *Assessing the Private Sector: Using Non-Government Resources to Strengthen Public Health Goals: Methodological Guidelines*. Boston, MA: Harvard School of Public Health.

Bhat, R. (1993). The private health care sector in India. In: Berman, P., Khan, M. (Eds). *Paying for India's Health Care*. New Delhi: Sage Publications.

Bhat, R. (1993). The private/public mix in health care in India. *Health Policy and Planning*, **8**(1), 43–56.

Bhat, R. (1996). Regulating the private health care sector: the case of the Indian Consumer Protection Act. *Health Policy and Planning*, **11**(3), 265–279.

Birdsall, N. (1994). Pragmatism, Robin Hood, and other themes: good government and social well-being in developing countries. In: Chen, L., Kleinman, A., Ware, N. (Eds). *Health and Social Change in International Perspective*. Boston, MA: Harvard University Press.

Chawla, M. (1995). *Dual Job Holdings by Government Physicians in Developing Countries*. Paper presented at the Regional Conference on Health Sector Reform in Asia, 22–25 May 1995. Manila, Philippines.

de Ferranti, D. (1984). Strategies for paying for health services in developing countries. *World Health Statistics Quarterly*, **37**(4), 428–442.

de Ferranti, D. (1985). *Paying for Health Services in Developing Countries: An Overview*. World Bank Staff Working Paper No. 721. Washington, DC: World Bank.

De Geynt, W. (1995). *Managing the Quality of Health Care in Developing Countries*. World Bank Technical Paper No. 258. Washington, DC: World Bank.

Donabedian, A. (1980). *Explorations in Quality: Assessment and Monitoring, Volume I: The Definition of Quality and Approaches to its Assessment*. Ann Arbor, MI: Health Administration Press.

Donabedian, A. (1982). *Explorations in Quality: Assessment and Monitoring, Volume II: The Criteria and Standards of Quality*. Ann Arbor, MI: Health Administration Press.

Donabedian, A. (1985). *Explorations in Quality: Assessment and Monitoring, Volume III: The Methods and Findings of Quality Assessment and Monitoring: An Illustrated Analysis*. Ann Arbor, MI: Health Administration Press.

Donabedian, A. (1988). The quality of care: how can it be assessed? *JAMA*, **260**(12), 1743–1748.

Dranove, D., White, W.D. (1994). Recent theory and evidence on competition in hospital markets. *Journal of Economic and Management Strategy*, **3**, 1.

Ellis, R., Chawla, M. (1993). *Public and Private Interactions in the Health Sector in Developing Countries*. Major Applied Research Paper No. 5. Bethesda, MD: Health Financing and Sustainability Project.

Feldstein, P. (1993). *Health Care Economics*. Albany, NY: Delmar Publications Inc.

Forsberg, B., Barros, F., Victora, C. (1992). Developing countries need more quality assurance: how health facility surveys can contribute. *Health Policy and Planning*, **7**(2), 193–196.

Frank, R., Salkever, D. (1994). Nonprofit organizations in the health sector. *Journal of Economic Perspectives*, **8**(4), 129–144.

Gabel, J., Redisch, V. (1979). Alternative physician payment methods: incentives, efficiency, and national health insurance. *Milbank Memorial Fund Quarterly*, **57**, 1.

Gani, A. (1990). Resources mobilization in the health sector. *Prisma*, **19**(6).

Griffin, C. (1989). *Strengthening Health Services in Developing Countries through the Private Sector*. IFC Discussion Paper No. 4. Washington, DC: World Bank.

Griffin, C. (1992). *Health Care in Asia: A Comparative Study of Cost and Financing*. Washington, DC: World Bank.

Hsiao, W. (1995). Abnormal economics in the health sector. In: Berman, P. (Ed.) *Health Sector Reform in Developing Countries: Making Health Development Sustainable*. Cambridge, MA: Harvard University Press, 161–182. Also published in *Health Policy*, **32**(1–3), 161–179.

Institute of Medicine. (1986). *For-Profit Enterprise in Health Care*. Washington, DC: National Academy Press.

Jeffers, J. (1989). Conceptual options for public–private partnerships in health care. *Privatization Review* (Spring).

Jeffers, J. (1990). Supply, demand and socio-economic factors influencing health policies. *Prisma*, **19**(6).

Ma, C. (1994). Health care payment systems: cost and quality incentives. *Journal of Economics and Management Strategy*, **3**, 1.

Mills, A. (1995). *Improving the Efficiency of Public Sector Health Services in Developing Countries: Bureaucratic versus Market Approaches*. London: London School of Tropical Medicine and Hygiene.

Musgrave, R. (1959). *The Theory of Public Finance*. New York: McGraw Hill.

Newbrander, W., Barnum, H., Kutzin, J. (1992). *Hospital Economics and Financing in Developing Countries*. Geneva: World Health Organization.

Newbrander, W., Parker, D. (1992). The public and private sectors in health: economic issues. *Int J Hlth Planning and Management*, **7**(1), 37–49.

Nichter, M. (1989). *Anthropology and International Health: South Asian Case Studies*. Boston, MA: Kluwer Academic Publishers.

Nittayaramphong, S., Tangcharoensathien, V. (1994). Thailand: private health care out of control? *Health Policy and Planning*, **9**(1), 31–40.

Normand, C., Weber, A. (1994). *Social Health Insurance: A Guidebook for Planning*. Geneva: World Health Organization.

Organization for Economic Cooperation and Development (OECD). (1990). *Health Care Systems in Transition*. Paris: OECD.

Paine, W., Tjam, S. (1988). *Hospitals and the Health Care Revolution*. Geneva: World Health Organization.

Parker, D., Newbrander, W. (1994). Tackling wastage and inefficiency in the health sector. *World Health Forum*, **15**(2), 107–113.

Racoveanu, N., Johansen, K. (1995). Technology for the continuous improvement of the quality of health care. *World Health Forum*, **16**(2), 138–144.

Rohde, E., Vishwanathan, H. (1995). *The Rural Private Practitioner*. New Delhi: Oxford University Press.

Rosenthal, G. (1970). Planning for health care — the choice of policies. In: Sheldon, A., Baker, F. (Eds). *Systems and Medical Care*. Boston: MIT Press.

Roth, G. (1987). *The Private Provision of Public Services in Developing Countries*. New York: Oxford University Press.

Saturno, P. (1995). Towards evaluation of the quality of care in health centres. *World Health Forum*, **16**(2), 145–150.

Shin, S., Yang, B. (1995). Change in service pattern under price control. *Korean Health Economic Review*, **1**(1), 53–73.

Solon, O., Gamboa, R., Schwartz, J., Herrin, A. (1991). *Health Sector Financing in the Philippines*, Vol. II. Research Triangle Institute and University of the Philippines School of Economics.

Solon, O., Gertler, P., Alabastro, S. (1995). *Insurance and Price Discrimination in the Market for Hospital Services in the Philippines*. Paper presented at the Asian Development Bank First Regional Conference on Health Sector Reform in Asia, May 22–25, 1995, Manila.

Spann, M. (1977). Public versus private provision of government services. In: Bortcherding, T. (Ed). *Budgets and Bureaucrats: The Sources of Government Growth.* Durham, NC: Duke University Press.

Vishwanathan, H., Rohde, J. (1990). *Diarrhoea in Rural India: A Nation-wide Study of Mothers and Practitioners.* New Delhi: Vision Books.

Wolf, C. (1988). *Markets or Governments: Choosing Between Implicit Alternatives.* Cambridge, MA: MIT.

World Bank. (1987). *Financing Health Services in Developing Countries: An Agenda for Reform.* Washington, DC: World Bank.

World Bank. (1993). *World Development Report 1993: Investing in Health.* New York: Oxford University Press.

World Bank. (1995). *World Development Report 1995: Workers in an Integrating World.* New York: Oxford University Press.

World Health Organization (WHO). (1991). *The Public/Private Mix in National Health Systems and the Role of Ministries of Health.* Report of a meeting held in Mexico, July 20–26, 1991. Geneva: WHO, Division of Strengthening of Health Services.

World Health Organization (WHO). (1994). *Evaluation of Recent Changes in the Financing of Health Services.* WHO Technical Report Series No. 829. Geneva: WHO.

Wouters, A. (1991). Essential national health research in developing countries: health-care financing and the quality of care. *Int J Hlth Planning and Management,* **6**(4), 253–271.

Yang, B. (1991). Health insurance in Korea: opportunities and challenges. *Health Policy and Planning,* **6**(2), 119–129.

Yang, B. (1995). *Health Care System of Korea: What Now and What in the Future?* Paper presented at the Asian Development Bank First Regional Conference on Health Sector Reform in Asia, May 22–25, 1995, Manila.

Glossary

Access: The ability of people to use health services unimpeded by financial or social constraints, or by lack of facilities or providers. Private sector provision of services is dependent on the existence of a market that generates adequate levels of demand even where the ability to pay is not an issue. Typically public action will be necessary to ensure access to services for populations in remote or sparsely populated areas. Policy options range from subsidy of supply (for example,, tax forgiveness for providers in underserved areas and direct guarantees of earnings) through contracts for services with private providers, to direct public provision.

Administrative Efficiency relates to administrative processes and procedures of systems or individual operating units, such as hospitals, which allow the services to be produced in the lowest-cost manner. These range from licensure, certification, and accreditation procedures of central agencies to the efficiency with which administrative matters are executed in connection with procurement, admission, billing, and payment mechanisms.

Allocative Efficiency relates to decisions on the mix of resources and where resources will be used to maximize output of services and promote equity. This decision deals with the desired mix of medical outputs consistent with medical need and consumer preferences, such as trade-offs between preventive and promotive health and curative health services, and specifically to the spread of medical technologies and types of medical interventions.

Budgets/Salary: Providers receive a fixed amount to operate their practice or facility for a given period. Budgets can be fixed by line-item or allow autonomy in use (global budget). Budgets can also finance a geographically-organized unit, like a district health authority, which could then pay providers using different methods. Individual providers in budget-based salary payment systems typically are paid a fixed compensation over a period of time regardless of volume of services provided.

Capitation: Providers are paid a fixed amount per person covered for a defined set of services over a defined period of time. Providers bear the risk if required services exceed the value of the payment, but also benefit if services delivered are less.

Case-based Payment: Providers are paid a fixed amount for a case or episode of illness. The amount is set in advance and may vary according to the type and severity of illness. The best known case-based payments systems use Diagnosis Related Groups (DRGs).

Continuous Quality Improvement (CQI) or Quality Improvement (QI) relates to the improvement of quality by examining the process by which care is provided and developing standardized practice patterns to narrow the variation of how care is provided. It generates treatment standards and protocols for providers to follow by giving them guidelines for dealing with patient conditions and suggesting options for care. Quality improvement uses the techniques of Total Quality Management (TQM).

Effectiveness: The financial incentives (particularly those associated with fees-for-service) for providers and the limited information available to patients increase the possibility that the most "profitable" services may not be the most effective. (For example, the widespread prescribing of antibiotics in lieu of oral rehydration salts in cases of infant diarrhea in many countries.) Public policies related to quality assurance, consumer protection, and regulations can all play a role in improving effectiveness in private production.

Efficiency and Costs: Although the private market incorporates incentives for more efficient production, market imperfections that result in higher costs (imperfect information, delegation of decision making, limited providers) will need to be directly addressed through public action. This is particularly important if the private sector is to have responsibility for an increasing share of service provision.

Equity relates to fairness in physical and financial access to a minimum package of health services. Concepts of equity involve value judgments. Physical access would include considerations of freedom of choice among alternative providers. Financial access would include considerations of universal entitlement to health insurance or other ways of removing financial barriers to receiving needed health services on behalf of the financially disadvantaged. Public options for addressing equity issues include strengthening private demand through subsidies for target populations, imposing service delivery obligations on private providers, and producing services publicly for these populations.

Fee-for-Service: Providers are paid a fee for each unit of service given. Units of service are typically defined as procedures, with wide variation across countries in the level of detail used to distinguish a unit of service. Prices per unit may be set in the market or negotiated.

Operational Efficiency relates to the classical economic concern for production efficiency in the use of resources relative to their costs in order to insure output is produced at minimum cost.

Quality Assurance (QA) involves assessing care already provided and taking action to improve care practices in the future. This is done by identifying the problems in health service delivery, analyzing those problems, and seeking to solve the problems to improve care provided in the future. This method seeks to identify "outliers" in medical practice and to correct those problems.

Quality of Care consists of the technical and interpersonal elements. Technical elements of quality are those aspects, such as the provider's behavior and skill in making interventions and applying technology. Interpersonal elements of quality are judged as good or bad according to how the care complies with the social norms, ethical standards, and client expectations. This term relates to the continuum of setting standards for the quality of inputs, the quality of processes involved in delivering services, and evaluating health outcomes continuously over time, such as Total Quality Management (TQM).

Structure–Process–Outcomes relates to the conceptual framework for assessing quality of care. Structure describes the attributes of the setting within which care is delivered. It is a static description of the relation of the structure to the actual process. The outcome of care is a measure of the patient's present and future health status attributable to the process of care. Process relates to the actual interaction between provider and client or patient. There is a causal link between the outcomes and what occurs during the process. Structure and outcomes are actually indirect means for assessing the process of care.

Systemic Efficiency (Scale Efficiency) relates to the overall organization of the health services delivery system and whether a system as a whole is producing services at the lowest cost. It includes such considerations as private and public sector mix, private and public sector cost sharing and integration, innovation, the degree of autonomy and self-sufficiency of the health system, referral system network, and other considerations.

Technical Efficiency relates to the mix of inputs (personnel, supplies, equipment, and facilities) which will produce a given output (health services). It is maximized when, for a given set of resources, the highest output possible is obtained. Alternatively, given a set level of output or services desired, it is maximized when the fewest possible inputs are used.

About the Asian Development Bank and Management Sciences for Health

The **Asian Development Bank (ADB)** is a regional multilateral development bank with 58 member countries. The ADB was created in 1966 to promote economic and social development in the region. In 1995, the Bank's lending reached $5.6 billion and its grant assistance was $145 million. As part of its mission, the ADB provides assistance to 36 developing member countries in Asia and the Pacific: Afghanistan, Bangladesh, Bhutan, Cambodia, China, Cook Islands, Fiji, Hong Kong, India, Indonesia, Kazakstan, Kiribati, Korea, Kyrgyzstan, Laos, Malaysia, Maldives, Marshall Islands, Micronesia, Mongolia, Myanmar, Nepal, Pakistan, Papua New Guinea, Philippines, Singapore, Solomon Islands, Sri Lanka, Taipei, Thailand, Tonga, Tuvalu, Vanuatu, Vietnam, and Western Samoa.

Recognizing the role of human resource development in overall economic progress, the ADB has a growing portfolio of activities to assist countries in making appropriate investments in the health sector. In recent years, as countries have expressed heightened interest in economic and sectoral reforms, the Bank has played a leadership role in sponsoring dialogue and research on health sector reform in the region. The ADB's address is the Asian Development Bank, Box 789, 1099 Manila, the Philippines; Telephone: 63-2-632-5531, Facsimile 63-2-636-2444.

Management Sciences for Health (MSH) is a private, nonprofit organization dedicated to closing the gap between what is known about public health problems and what is done to solve them. Since its founding in 1971, MSH has collaborated with health policy-makers and health care managers throughout the world to improve the quality of health and population services and to make these services accessible and affordable for all.

During its 25-year history, MSH has assisted public- and private-sector health and population programs in over 100 countries. MSH has provided technical assistance, conducted training, carried out applied research, and developed systems for use in health program management. MSH has managed major projects dealing with health financing; health care and hospital services and management; family planning and reproductive health services; development of national health policies; procurement, management, and rational use of pharmaceuticals; and training managers around the world. Its 200 technical and management staff from 36 nations is based in Boston and Washington, DC, with field offices throughout the world.

The MSH's Health Financing Program has helped government policy-makers and health program managers develop and implement practical financing strategies to use existing resources efficiently, generate additional resources, and achieve sustainability. It has facilitated health sector reform through cost sharing, health insurance, privatization, sustainability, and decentralization. The program's address is Management Sciences for Health, Health Financing Program, 165 Allandale Road, Boston, Massachusetts 02130-3400, USA; Telephone: 1-617-524-7799, Facsimile: 1-617-524-2825, e-mail: hfp@msh.org.

Author Index

Note: page numbers in *italics* refer to figures and tables

Subject Index

Note: page numbers in *italics* refer to figures and tables

Indexes compiled by Jill Halliday